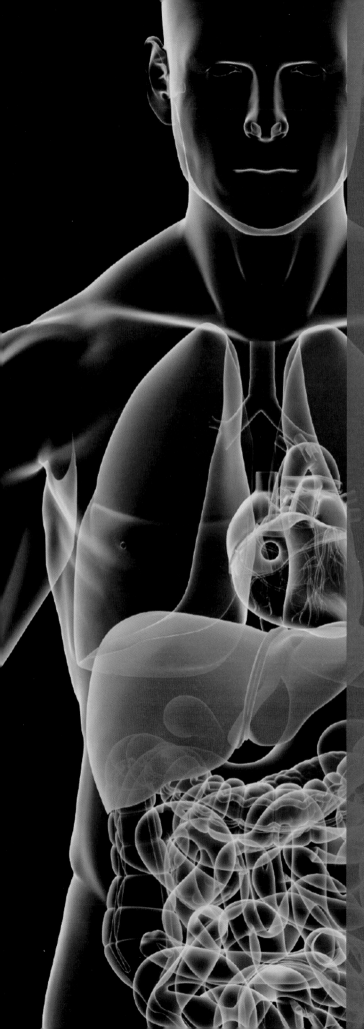

Hepatology
at a Glance

Deepak Joshi
Consultant Hepatologist
King's College Hospital
London, UK

Geri Keane
Clinical Research Fellow
Institute for Liver and Digestive Health
University College London
London, UK

Alison Brind
Consultant Gastroen
Hepatology
University Hospital o
Stoke on Trent, UK

D1354850

bsg

BRITISH SOCIETY OF
GASTROENTEROLOGY

WILEY Blackwell

This edition first published 2015 © 2015 by John Wiley & Sons, Ltd.

Registered Office
John Wiley & Sons, Ltd, The Atrium, Southern Gate, Chichester, West Sussex, PO19 8SQ, UK

Editorial Offices
9600 Garsington Road, Oxford, OX4 2DQ, UK
The Atrium, Southern Gate, Chichester, West Sussex, PO19 8SQ, UK
350 Main Street, Malden, MA 02148-5020, USA

For details of our global editorial offices, for customer services and for information about how to apply for permission to reuse the copyright material in this book please see our website at www.wiley.com/wiley-blackwell

Library of Congress Cataloging-in-Publication Data

Joshi, Deepak, author.
  Hepatology at a glance / Deepak Joshi, Geri Keane, Alison Brind.
    p. ; cm.
  Includes index.
  ISBN 978-1-118-75939-4 (pbk.)
  I. Keane, Margaret G. (Margaret Geraldine), author.   II. Brind, Alison, author.   III. Title.
  [DNLM: 1. Liver Diseases. WI 700]
  RC845
  616.3'62–dc23

                                    2014040281

A catalogue record for this book is available from the British Library.

Wiley also publishes its books in a variety of electronic formats. Some content that appears in print may not be available in electronic books.

Cover image: iStock/ © Eraxion

Set in 9.5/11.5pt Minion by SPi Publisher Services, Pondicherry, India
Printed and bound in Singapore by Markono Print Media Pte Ltd

1   2015

Contents

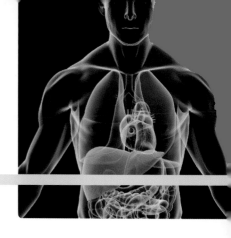

Preface

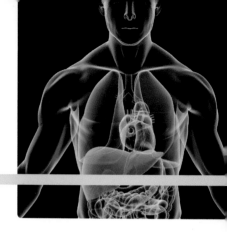

Hepatology is a rapidly growing specialty with increasing emphasis within the medical curriculum requiring an 'at a Glance' of its own. We have integrated core principles of basic science, pathophysiology, treatments and management algorithms into a single easy-to-use text. As such, it can be used by medical students throughout their training, junior doctors entering the field of hepatology and also by allied health care professionals with an interest in hepatology.

As with other *at a Glance* publications, *Hepatology at a Glance* is based around a two-page spread for each main topic, with colour figures and text complementing each other to give an overview of a topic. Case studies based on some of the most commonly encountered presentations in hepatology are included. The book covers all the core elements of hepatology and its major diseases; further reading suggestions are included for more in-depth study. The self-assessment MCQs are designed as a single best response in keeping with the specialty certificate examination in gastroenterology.

The publishers of '*at Glance*' approached the education committee of the British Society of Gastroenterology (BSG) who selected the authors. We should like to thank the BSG for their support and the opportunity to contribute to the literature with this innovative publication. In addition, we would like to thank all our colleagues who took the time to review each chapter and ensure the content was of the highest standard. We also thank the staff at Wiley Blackwell, without whom we would not have been able to produce this new and exciting first edition.

Deepak Joshi
Geri Keane
Alison Brind

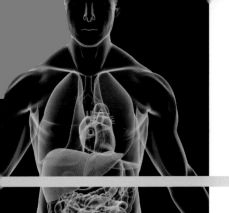

Acknowledgements

Dr Kosh Agarwal, King's College Hospital, London
Dr Ahmir Ahmad, Imperial College, London
Professor GP Aithal, Queens Medical Centre, Nottingham
Dr Zahir Amin, University College London Hospitals, London
Dr Quentin Anstee, Freeman Hospital, Newcastle
Dr Adrian Bateman, Southampton General Hospital, Southampton
Dr Mike Brown, University College London Hospitals, and Hospital for Tropical Diseases, London
Dr Mike Chapman, University College London Hospitals, London
Professor Anil Dhawan, King's College Hospital, London
Dr Catherine Edwards, Torbay Hospital, Torquay
Dr Michael Heneghan, King's College Hospital, London
Dr Gavin Johnson, University College London Hospitals, London
Dr TuVinh Luong, Royal Free Hospital, London
Professor John O'Grady, King's College Hospital, London
Dr Steve Pereira, University College London Hospitals, London
Professor Massimo Pinzani, UCL Institute for Liver and Digestive Health, London
Dr Samantha Read, University College London Hospitals, London
Dr Andrew Rochford, Barts Health, London
Dr Debbie Shawcross, King's College Hospital, London
Dr Nick Sheron, University Hospital, Southampton
Dr Douglas Thorburn, Royal Free Hospital, London
Dr Paul Trembling, Royal Free Hospital, London
Dr Manolis Tsochatzis, Royal Free Hospital, London
Dr Sumita Verma, Brighton and Sussex Medical School, Brighton
Dr George Webster, University College London Hospitals, London.

Figure sources

Anstee QM, Targer G, Day CP. Progression of NAFLD to diabetes mellitus, cardiovascular disease or cirrhosis. *Nature Reviews Gastroenterology and Hepatology* 2013;10:330–44.

Babor TF, Higgins-Biddle JC, Saunders JB, Monteiro JG. *AUDIT: Guidelines for Use in Primary Care*, 2nd edn. WHO, 2001.

Beeching N, Gill G (eds) *Lecture Notes: Tropical Medicine,* 7th edn. Wiley Blackwell, 2014.

Bellomo R, Ronco C, Kellum JA, Mehta RL, Palevsky P; Acute Dialysis Quality Initiative workgroup. Acute renal failure – definition, outcome measures, animal models, fluid therapy and information technology needs: the Second International Consensus Conference of the Acute Dialysis Quality Initiative (ADQI) Group. *Critical Care* 2004;8(4):R204–12.

Dooley JS, Lok A, Burroughs AK, Heathcote J (eds) *Sherlock's Diseases of the Liver and Biliary System*, 12th edn. Blackwell Publishing, 2011.

EASL–EORTC Clinical Practice Guidelines: Management of hepatocellular carcinoma. *European Journal of Cancer* 2012;48: 599–641.

Friedman SL. Mechanisms of disease: Mechanisms of hepatic fibrosis and therapeutic implications. *Nature Clinical Practice Gastroenterology and Hepatology* 2004;1:98–105.

Friedman SL. Mechanisms of hepatic fibrogenesis. *Gastroenterology* 2008;134(6):1655–669.

García-Martinez R, Córdoba J. Acute-on-chronic liver failure: the brain. *Current Opinion in Critical Care* 2011;17:177–83.

Gleeson D, Heneghan MA. British Society of Gastroenterology (BSG) guidelines for management of autoimmune hepatitis. *Gut* 2011;60:1611–29.

Goossens N, Joshi D, O'Grady J. Image of the month. Digital clubbing in association with hepatopulmonary syndrome. *Hepatology* 2010;53(1):365–6.

Hajarizadeh B, Grebely J, Dore GJ. Epidemiology and natural history of HCV infection. *Nature Clinical Practice Gastroenterology and Hepatology* 2013;10(9):553–62.

Joshi D, Belgaumkar A, Ratnayake V, Quaglia A, Austin D. A case of hepatomegaly. *Postgraduate Medical Journal* 2007;83(984):e2.

Keane MG, Marlow NJ, Pereira SP. Novel endoscopic approaches in the diagnosis and management of biliary strictures. *Prime Reports* 2014;32(5):570–8.

Keane MG, Pereira SP. Improving the detection and treatment of liver cancer. *The Practitioner* 2013;257:21–6.

Keshav S, Bailey A. *The Gastrointestinal System at a Glance*, 2nd edn. John Wiley & Sons Ltd, 2013.

Mieli-Vergani G, Vergani D. Autoimmune hepatitis. *Nature Reviews Gastroenterology and Hepatology* 2011;8:320–7.

Papastergiou V, Tsochatzis E, Burroughs A. Non-invasive assessment of liver fibrosis. *Annals of Gastroenterology* 2012;25:218–31.

Skipworth JRA, Keane MG, Pereira SP. Update on the management of cholangiocarcinoma. *Digestive Diseases* 2014;32(5):570–8.

Utzschneider KM, Kowdley KV. Hereditary hemochromatosis and diabetes mellitus: implications for clinical practice. *Nature Reviews in Endocrinology* 2010;6:26–33.

Watt KDS, Pedersen RA, Kremers WK, Heimbach JK, Charlton MR. Evolution of causes and risk factors for mortality post-liver transplant: results of the NIDDK long-term follow-up study. *American Journal of Transplantation* 2010:6;1420–7.

Zarrinpar A, Busuttil RW. Liver transplantation: past, present and future. *Nature Clinical Practice Gastroenterology and Hepatology* 2013;10:434–40.

List of abbreviations

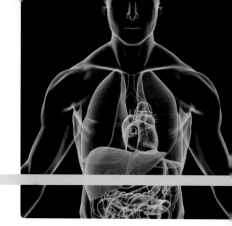

A1AT	α1-antitrypsin deficiency		CREST	(syndrome of) calcinosis, Raynaud's phenomenon, oesophageal dysmotility, sclerodactyly and telangiectasia
ABG	arterial blood gas			
ACE	angiotensin-converting enzyme			
ACR	acute cellular rejection		CRP	C-reactive protein
ADR	adverse drug reaction		CT	computed tomography
AFB	acid-fast bacillus		CVD	cardiovascular disease
AFLP	acute fatty liver of pregnancy		CYP	cytochrome P450
AFP	alpha-fetoprotein		DAA	directly acting antiviral
AIH	autoimmune hepatitis		DBD	donor after brain death
AKI	acute kidney injury		DCD	donor after cardiac death
ALD	alcohol-related liver disease		DEXA	dual-energy X-ray absorptiometry
ALF	acute liver failure		DF	Maddrey's discriminate function
ALP	alkaline phosphatase		DIC	disseminated intravascular coagulation
ALPPS	associating liver partition with portal vein ligation for staged hepatectomy		DILI	drug-induced liver injury
			DLCO	carbon monoxide diffusing capacity
ALT	alanine transaminase		EASL	European Association for the Study of the Liver
AMA	anti-mitochondrial antibody		EBL	endoscopic band ligation
ANA	antinuclear antibody		EBV	Epstein–Barr virus
AP	acute pancreatitis		ECM	extracellular matrix
APTT	activated partial thromboplastin time		EHPVO	extrahepatic portal vein obstruction
ARFI	acoustic radiation force impulse		EN	enteral nutrition
ASMA	anti-smooth muscle antibody		EPO	erythropoietin
AASLD	American Association for the Study of Liver Diseases		ERCP	endoscopic retrograde cholangiopancreatography
AST	aspartate transaminase		EUS	endoscopic ultrasound
ATP	adenosine triphosphate		FBC	full blood count
AUDIT	Alcohol Use Disorders Identification Test		FDG	2-fluoro-2-deoxy-D-glucose
BAT	biliary atresia		FDP	fibrinogen degradation product
BMI	body mass index		FHF	fulminant hepatic failure
BNP	brain natriuretic peptide		FHVP	free hepatic vein pressure
BRIC	benign recurrent intrahepatic cholestasis		FLR	future liver remnant
BRTO	balloon-occluded retrograde transvenous obliteration		FNA	fine needle aspiration
			FNH	focal nodular hyperplasia
BSEP	bile salt export protein		GCS	Glasgow Coma Score
cAMP	cyclic adenosine monophosphate		GCSF	granulocyte colony-stimulating factor
CC	cholangiocarcinoma		GFR	glomerular filtration rate
CF	cystic fibrosis		GGT	gamma-glutamyltransferase
CFLD	cystic fibrosis-related liver disease		GHS	Glasgow Hepatitis Score
CHBV	chronic hepatitis B virus infection		GLP	glucagon-like peptide
CIWA-Ar	Clinical Institute Withdrawal Assessment Scale		GV	gastric varices
CKD	chronic kidney disease		HAART	highly active antiretroviral therapy
CLD	chronic liver disease		HAT	hepatic artery thrombosis
CLD	coagulopathy in liver disease		HAV	hepatitis A virus
CMV	cytomegalovirus		HBIG	hepatitis B immunoglobulin
CNI	calcineurin inhibitor		HBsAg	hepatitis B surface antigen
coA	coenzyme A		HCC	hepatocellular carcinoma
COPD	chronic obstructive pulmonary disease		HCV	hepatitis C virus

HDL	high density lipoprotein	OGD	oesophago-gastro-duodenoscopy
HDU	high dependency unit	ONS	oral nutritional supplement
H&E	haematoxylin and eosin	OTC	over-the-counter
HE	hepatic encephalopathy	OV	oesophageal varices
HELLP	haemolysis, elevated liver enzymes, low platelets (syndrome)	PAH	pulmonary arterial hypertension
		PAS	periodic acid–Schiff
HEV	hepatitis E virus	PBC	primary biliary cirrhosis
HH	hereditary haemochromatosis	PBG	porphobilinogen
HIDA	hepatobiliary iminodiacetic acid	PCWP	pulmonary capillary wedge pressure
HMG	3-hydroxy-3-methylglutaryl	PDAC	pancreatic ductal adenocarcinoma
HPS	hepato-pulmonary syndrome	PDGF	platelet derived growth factor
HRS	hepato-renal syndrome	PEG-IFN	pegylated interferon
HSC	hepatic stellate cell	PELD	Paediatric End-stage Liver Disease
HSV	herpes simplex virus	PET	positron emission tomography
HVPG	hepatic venous pressure gradient	PFIC	progressive familial intrahepatic cholestasis
IAIHG	International Autoimmune Hepatitis Group	PHT	portal hypertension
IBD	inflammatory bowel disease	PN	parenteral nutrition
ICP	intrahepatic cholestasis of pregnancy	PNET	pancreatic neuroendocrine tumour
IFALD	intestinal failure-associated liver disease	POPH	porto-pulmonary hypertension
Ig	immunoglobulin	PPAR	peroxisome proliferator-activated receptor
IGF	insulin-like growth factor	PSC	primary sclerosing cholangitis
IL	interleukin	PT	prothrombin time
INR	international normalised ratio	PVT	portal vein hepatitis
IPMN	intraductal papillary mucinous neoplasm	RBBB	right bundle branch block
ITU	intensive treatment unit	ROS	reactive oxidative species
IV	intravenous	RUQ	right upper quadrant
IVC	inferior vena cava	SAAG	serum ascites albumin gradient
IVDU	intravenous drug user	SADQ	Severity of Alcohol Dependence Questionnaire
IVPD	intrapulmonary vascular dilatation		
KF	Kayser–Fleischer	SBT	Sengstaken–Blakemore tube
LC	liver cytosolic	SBP	spontaneous bacterial peritonitis
LDH	lactate dehydrogenase	SCA	serous cyst adenoma
LDL	low density lipoprotein	SCC	secondary sclerosing cholangitis
LFT	liver function test	SEMS	self-expanding metal stent
LKM	liver kidney microsomal	SMA	smooth muscle antibody
LPS	lipopolysaccharide	SOD	sphincter of Oddi dysfunction
LT	liver transplantation	SSRI	selective serotonin reuptake inhibitor
LVP	large volume paracentesis	SVR	sustained virologic response
MCN	mucinous cystadenoma	TB	tuberculosis
MELD	Model for End-stage Liver Disease	TEG	thromboelastography
MMP	matrix metalloproteinase	TF	tissue factor
MMSE	Mini Mental State Examination	TGF	transforming growth factor
mPAP	mean pulmonary artery pressure	TIMMP	tissue inhibitors of matrix metalloproteinase
MR	magnetic resonance	TIPS	transjugular intrahepatic portosystemic shunt
MRCP	magnetic resonance cholangiopancreatography	TLR	Toll-like receptor
MRE	magnetic resonance elastography	TNF	tumour necrosis factor
MRI	magnetic resonance imaging	TPA	tissue plasminogen activator
MRP	multidrug resistance protein	TPMT	thiopurine methlytransferase
MSM	men who have sex with men	UDCA	ursodeoxycholic acid
NAC	N-acetylcysteine	U&E	urea and electrolytes
NAFLD	non-alcoholic fatty liver disease	UGT	uridine diphosphoglucuronate-glucuronosyltransferase
NASH	non-alcoholic steatohepatitis		
NCPF	non-cirrhotic portal fibrosis	ULN	upper limit of normal
NCPH	non-cirrhotic portal hypertension	US	ultrasound
NF-κB	nuclear factor κB	VEGF	vascular endothelial growth factor
NODM	new onset diabetes mellitus	VLDL	very low density lipoprotein
NSAID	non-steroidal anti-inflammatory drug	vWf	von Willebrand factor
NSBB	non-selective beta-blocker	WCC	white cell count
OCP	oral contraceptive pill	WHVP	wedged hepatic vein pressure

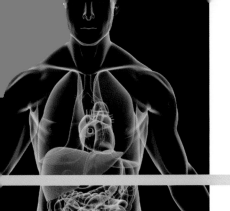

How to use your revision guide

Features contained within your revision guide

The overview page gives a summary of the topics covered in each part.

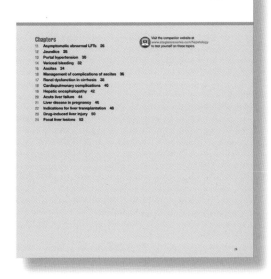

Clinical scenarios **Part 3**

Each topic is presented in a double-page spread with clear, easy-to-follow diagrams supported by succinct explanatory text.

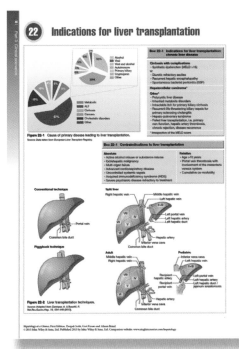

The anytime, anywhere textbook

Wiley E-Text

Your book is also available to purchase as a **Wiley E-Text: Powered by VitalSource** version – a digital, interactive version of this book which you own as soon as you download it.

Your **Wiley E-Text** allows you to:

Search Save time by finding terms and topics instantly in your book, your notes, even your whole library (once you've downloaded more textbooks)

Note and Highlight Colour code, highlight and make digital notes right in the text so you can find them quickly and easily

Organize Keep books, notes and class materials organized in folders inside the application

Share Exchange notes and highlights with friends, classmates and study groups

Upgrade Your textbook can be transferred when you need to change or upgrade computers

The **Wiley E-Text** version will also allow you to copy and paste any photograph or illustration into assignments, presentations and your own notes.

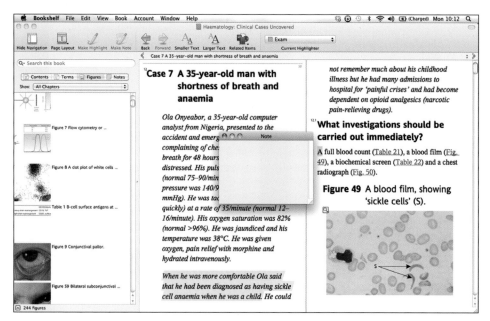

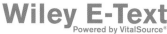

To access your Wiley E-Text:

- Visit **www.vitalsource.com/software/bookshelf/downloads** to download the Bookshelf application to your computer, laptop, tablet or mobile device.
- Open the Bookshelf application on your computer and register for an account.
- Follow the registration process.

CourseSmart

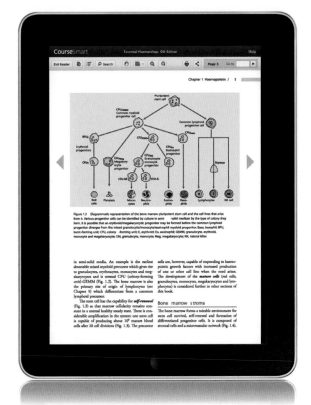

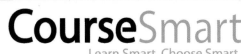

About the companion website

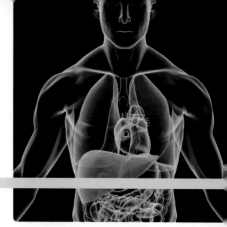

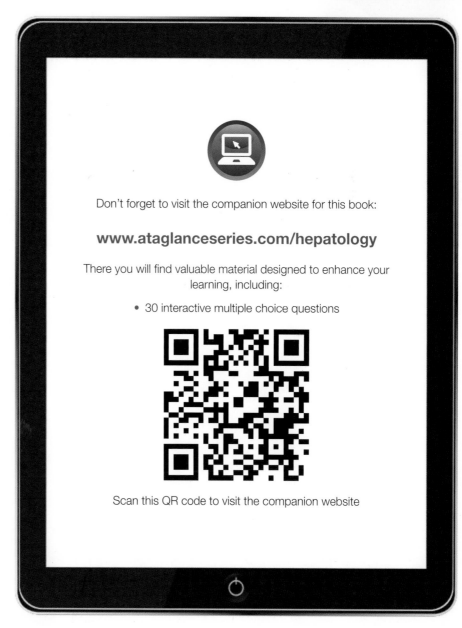

Don't forget to visit the companion website for this book:

www.ataglanceseries.com/hepatology

There you will find valuable material designed to enhance your learning, including:

- 30 interactive multiple choice questions

Scan this QR code to visit the companion website

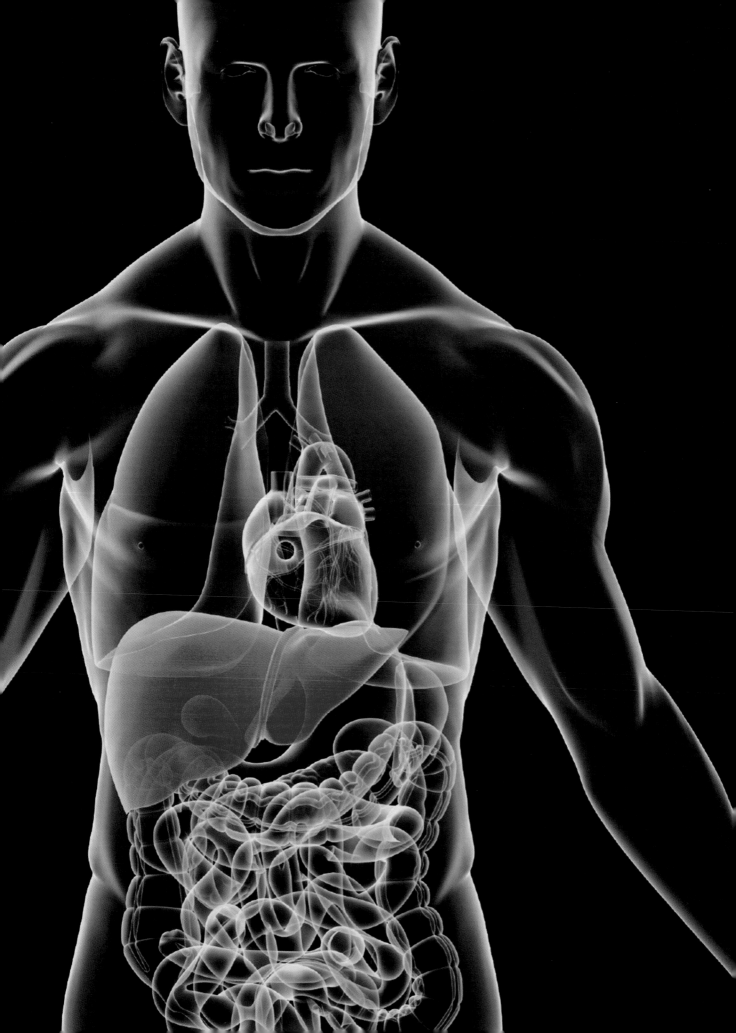

Basics

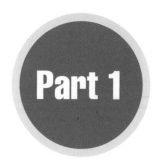

Chapters

Visit the companion website at
www.ataglanceseries.com/hepatology
to test yourself on these topics

Liver and biliary anatomy and structure

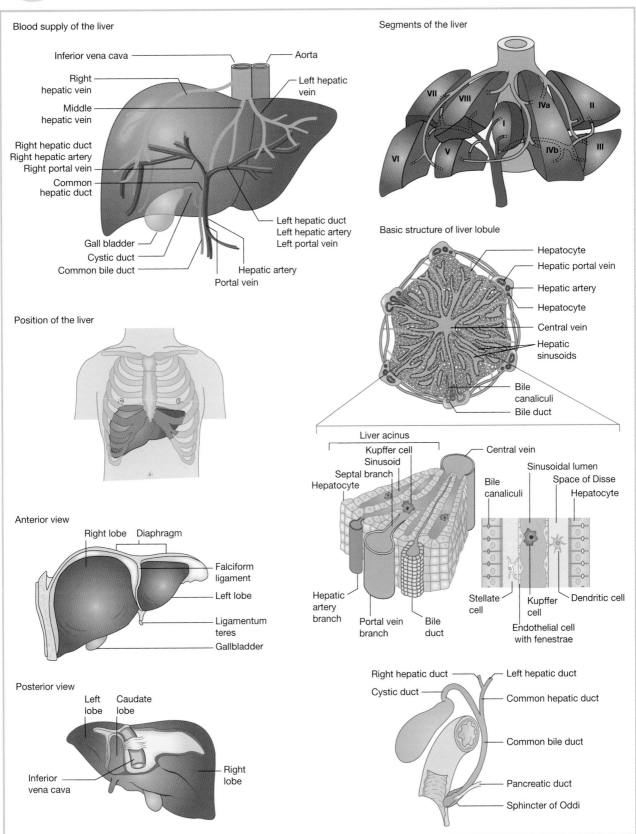

Blood supply of the liver

Inferior vena cava
Aorta
Right hepatic vein
Left hepatic vein
Middle hepatic vein
Right hepatic duct
Right hepatic artery
Right portal vein
Common hepatic duct
Left hepatic duct
Left hepatic artery
Left portal vein
Gall bladder
Cystic duct
Common bile duct
Hepatic artery
Portal vein

Position of the liver

Anterior view

Right lobe   Diaphragm
Falciform ligament
Left lobe
Ligamentum teres
Gallbladder

Posterior view

Left lobe   Caudate lobe
Inferior vena cava
Right lobe

Segments of the liver

VII   VIII   IVa   II
I
VI   V   IVb   III

Basic structure of liver lobule

Hepatocyte
Hepatic portal vein
Hepatic artery
Hepatocyte
Central vein
Hepatic sinusoids
Bile canaliculi
Bile duct

Liver acinus

Kupffer cell
Sinusoid
Septal branch
Hepatocyte
Central vein
Bile canaliculi
Sinusoidal lumen
Space of Disse
Hepatocyte
Hepatic artery branch
Portal vein branch
Bile duct
Stellate cell
Kupffer cell
Dendritic cell
Endothelial cell with fenestrae

Right hepatic duct
Left hepatic duct
Cystic duct
Common hepatic duct
Common bile duct
Pancreatic duct
Sphincter of Oddi

Hepatology at a Glance, First Edition. Deepak Joshi, Geri Keane and Alison Brind.
© 2015 John Wiley & Sons, Ltd. Published 2015 by John Wiley & Sons, Ltd. Companion website: www.ataglanceseries.com/hepatology

Development

The liver begins as a hollow endodermal bud from the foregut (duodenum) in the third week of gestation. The bud then separates into the hepatic and biliary components. The hepatic part contains bipotential progenitor cells that differentiate into hepatocytes or ductal cells, which form the early biliary duct plates. These rapidly proliferating cells penetrate adjacent mesodermal tissue (septum transversum) and are met by a growing vascular capillary plexus from the vitelline and umbilical veins, which form the sinusoids. The gallbladder and extra-hepatic bile ducts are formed from the connection of these proliferating cells and the foregut. The liver structure is formed by epithelial liver cords that differentiate into hepatocytes, bile canalilculi and hepatic ducts. Bile flows from the 12th week. Kupffer cells are derived from circulating monocytes while hepatic stellate cells are derived from submesothelial cells.

Macro liver and biliary anatomy

The liver is the largest internal organ, weighing 1.2–1.5 kg. It is surrounded by a capsule of connective tissue (Glisson's capsule). It is situated in the right upper quadrant, shielded by the ribs and moves with respiration due to attachment to the diaphragm. The upper border lies at the level of the nipples/fifth rib. The liver contains two lobes; the larger **right** lobe that also contains the **caudate** (posterior surface) and **quadrate** (inferior surface) lobes, and the **left** lobe. The two lobes are separated anteriorly by the **falciform ligament**, posteriorly by the **ligamentum venosum** and inferiorly by the **ligamentum teres**. The **middle hepatic vein** runs between the right and left lobes. The liver can be further divided into eight segments based upon the division of the right middle and left hepatic veins.

The **right** and **left hepatic biliary ducts** exit the liver and unite at the hilum to form the **common hepatic duct**. The **gallbladder** is situated above the transverse colon. The body of the gallbladder narrows at the neck before becoming the cystic duct. The **cystic duct** then joins to form the **common bile duct**. The common bile duct lies anterior to the portal vein and passes behind the first part of the duodenum before entering the second part of the duodenum. It joins the pancreatic duct to form a common channel, the **ampulla of Vater**. In the duodenum the ampulla forms a membranous bulge, the major duodenal papilla. The **sphincter of Oddi** comprises thickened longitudinal and circular muscle fibres and is the duodenal component of the common bile duct. It contracts intermittently, controlling the release of bile.

Blood and lymphatic supply

The liver has a dual blood supply from the **portal vein** and the **hepatic artery**. Approximately 25% of the liver's blood supply is supplied by the hepatic artery, which originates from the **coeliac axis**. The portal vein provides 75% of the liver's blood supply and returns venous blood from the gastrointestinal tract and spleen. Both vessels enter the liver through the **porta hepatis (liver hilum)**. Inside the hilum, the portal vein and hepatic artery divide into the right and left branches supplying their respective lobes before being distributed to the segments and flows into the **sinusoids** via the portal tracts. Blood leaves the sinusoids and then enters tributories of the hepatic veins (middle, right and left) before entering the **inferior vena cava**. The caudate lobe receives a separate blood supply from the portal vein and hepatic artery while its hepatic vein drains directly into the inferior vena cava.

The **cystic artery** provides the gallbladder's blood supply while drainage is via the **cystic vein**. The majority of the blood supply to the bile ducts is from the **retroduodenal and right hepatic arteries**.

Lymph collects in the portal tracts and enters larger vessels before entering the hepatic ducts.

Micro liver structure

Liver lobes are made up of microscopic units called lobules which are hexangonal in shape. The **acinus** is the functional structural unit of the liver. It is an elliptical unit with a **portal triad** at the centre, a **central vein** at each pole and has three zones:
- Zone 1: *periportal*. Contains most oxygenated blood. Most susceptible to damage from toxins entering liver. Performs majority of metabolic activity.
- Zone 2: *midzone*.
- Zone 3: *centrilobular*. Closest to central vein. Most susceptible to ischaemic damage.

Hepatocytes are arranged in cords which radiate out from the central vein. Blood-filled sinusoids form networks between the hepatocytes which are lined with a fenestrated endothelium. Between the hepatocytes and **sinusoidal endothelial cells** is the **perisinusoidal space of Disse** which contains **Kupffer cells** and **hepatic stellate cells**. Kupffer cells have phagocytic capacity and are the resident hepatc macrophages. Hepatic stellate cells store vitamin A and produce collagen in response to injury. Microvilli are seen at the sinusoidal surface and increase the surface area for transfer of oxygen, nutrients, and so on, between blood in the sinusoids and hepatocytes. **Bile canaliculi** are formed by a channel between two surfaces of hepatocytes and are sealed by **zonulae occludentes**. They join to form bile ductules in the portal tracts by opening into **canals of Hering**. These canals drain bile into the biliary ductule of the portal tracts.

Anatomical abnormalities
Riedel's lobe

This is an anatomical variation characterised by a downward projection of the right lobe of the liver. It moves with respiration and can descend as far down as the right iliac fossa. It is more common in women more but is usually asymptomatic.

2 Liver metabolism and function

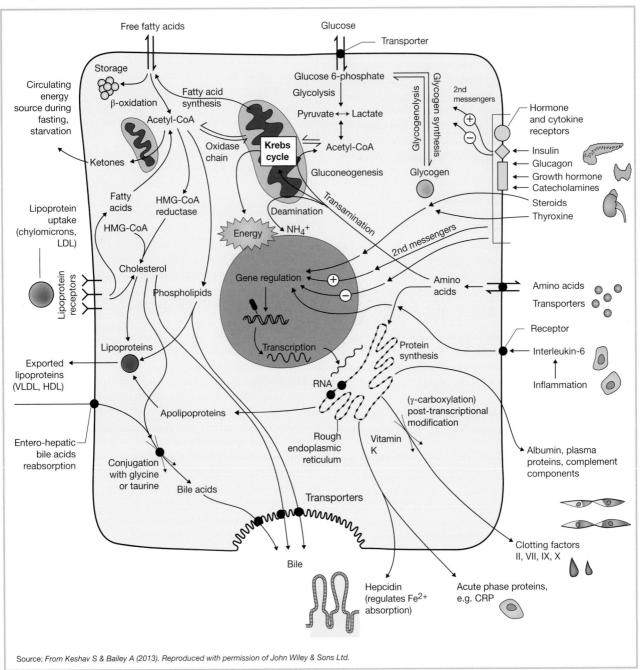

Source: *From Keshav S & Bailey A (2013). Reproduced with permission of John Wiley & Sons Ltd.*

Metabolism

The liver is a highly complex organ with regards to metabolic function. Understanding the liver's basic metabolic function allows one to recognise how patients present with both acute and chronic liver disease. At present, no artificial devices exist that can mimic the liver's metabolic function.

Carbohydrates

The liver performs a key role in glucose production and homeostasis. It is the major store of glucose in the body, in the form of glycogen. In the fasting state, glycogen can be broken by glycogenolysis, in periportal hepatocytes, to maintain normoglycaemia. Gluconeogenesis produces glucose and sources include lactate,

Hepatology at a Glance, First Edition. Deepak Joshi, Geri Keane and Alison Brind.
© 2015 John Wiley & Sons, Ltd. Published 2015 by John Wiley & Sons, Ltd. Companion website: www.ataglanceseries.com/hepatology

pyruvate, amino acids and glycerol. Ketone bodies and fatty acids are utilised in prolonged starvation. Glycolysis involves the conversion of glucose-6-phosphate to pyruvate. Pyruvate is converted to lactate under anaerobic conditions by the enzyme lactate dehydrogenase (LDH) or to acetyl-coA (coenzyme A).

Lipids

Dietary lipids are transported as chylomicrons and are taken up into the liver. The liver metabolises these lipids to produce cholesterol, phospholipids, triglycerides and free fatty acids. These lipids are then re-assembled as lipoproteins before being transported around the body. Lipoproteins are created from apolipoproteins and hydrophobic lipids. Important lipoproteins include very low density lipoproteins (VLDL), high density lipoproteins (HDL) and low density lipoproteins (LDL).

Protein

Amino acids absorbed from the small intestine enter the liver via the portal vein. Hepatocytes transport amino acids through sodium dependent and -independent systems. Amino acids are then either transaminated or deaminated to keto-acids which are metabolised via the Krebs or citric acid cycle.

Hormones and vitamins

Insulin, glucagon, oestrogens, corticosteroids and growth hormone are catabolised in the liver. Vitamin D metabolism also occurs in the liver (conversion of cholecalciferol to 25-hydroxy-cholecalciferol).

Drug metabolism

Drugs are metabolised within the liver through three distinct phases:

- *Phase I reactions.* Drugs undergo reduction or oxidation predominately through the cytochrome P450 (CYP) superfamily predominantly within the endoplasmic reticulum. CYP1, CYP2, CYP3, and in particular CYP3A4 are integral in drug metabolism.
- *Phase II reactions.* Drugs or their metabolites are conjugated to glucoronic acid, sulfate, acetate, glycine, glutathione or a methyl group. Conjugation occurs within in the cytoplasm of hepatocytes via uridine diphosphoglucuronate-glucuronosyltransferase (UGT), sulfotransferases and glutathione S-transferase. Conjugates are more soluble.
- *Phase III reactions.* Drugs and their products are transported into bile. Biliary excretion is mediated by adenosine triphosphate (ATP) dependent transporters.

Synthesis
Protein

The most important protein produced by the liver is albumin. 10–12 g albumin is produced daily. Albumin helps transport bilirubin, hormones and fatty acids, all of which are water-insoluble. Hypoalbuminaemia is common in chronic liver disease but can also occur in patients with severe illness, severe sepsis or where protein is being lost from the bowel (protein losing enteropathy) or via the kidneys (nephrotic syndrome). Gammaglobulins are not produced in the liver. Other protein synthesised in the liver include transport proteins transferrin and caeruloplasmin, α1-antitrypsin, alpha-feto proteins, α2-macroglobulin, complement, fibrinogen and ferritin. Liver proteins are also acute phase proteins and are released from the liver when hepatic injury occurs (e.g. C-reactive protein, ferritin, hepcidin, complement, caeruloplasmin and fibrinogen).

The liver also produces specific coagulation factors (II, V, VII, IX and X). This mechanism is through a vitamin K dependent gamma-carboxylation.

Bile

Approximately 600 mL alkaline bile is produced daily. It consists of:

- Primary bile acids: cholic acid and chenodeoxycholic acid (formed from cholesterol);
- Secondary bile acids: deoxycholic and lithocholic acid;
- Phospholipids;
- Cholesterol;
- Bilirubin (see Chapter 7);
- Conjugated drugs and endogenous waste products; and
- Na^+, Cl^-, $HCO3^-$, copper.

Bile acids

Bile acid synthesis is via a negative feedback loop. Bile acids are synthesised by either 7α-hydroxylation of cholesterol by CYP7A1 (classic pathway) resulting in cholic acid and chenodeoxycholic acid or through CYP27 (alternate pathway) which results in the synthesis of chenodeoxycholic acid. Bile acids are conjugated in the liver to amino acids glycine or taurine and prevent precipitation and allow absorption in the terminal ileum. Bile acids are excreted into the biliary canaliculi using ATP stimulated transporters and then stored in the gallbladder. Unconjugated bile acids are secreted via the bile salt export protein (BSEP). Bile acids are reabsorbed in the terminal ileum and then enter the portal venous system before being taken up by hepatocytes.

Ammonia

Ammonia is created following the degradation of amino acids and is then converted to urea before excretion via the kidneys. Ammonia that is not broken down into urea is synthesised into glutamine.

Lipids
Cholesterol

Cholestrol is predominantly synthesised in the liver. It is found in cell membranes and is a precursor of bile acids and steroid hormones. Cholesterol is stored in the liver as cholesterol ester. It is excreted from the liver in bile. Synthesis is increased following biliary obstruction, terminal ileal resection and corticosteroids. Synthesis is decreased by statins (inhibit conversion of 3-hydroxy-3-methylglutaryl (HMG) to mevalonate by inhibiting HMG CoA reductase), fasting, fibrates and bile salts.

Phospholipids

Phospholipids are an important constituent of cell membranes. The most abundant is lecithin (phosphatidyl choline). They are secreted into the bile.

Immunological function

Blood arriving in the liver via the portal vein is rich in bacteria, other foreign pathogens and antigens. Kupffer cells phagocytose and degrade these foreign bodies. The liver provides an important component of the innate immune system. It secretes chemokines and cytokines including interleukins (IL) and tumour necrosis factor (TNF). T- and B-cell lymphocytes also interact within the liver. The liver therefore provides an important immunological barrier.

3 Coagulation in liver disease

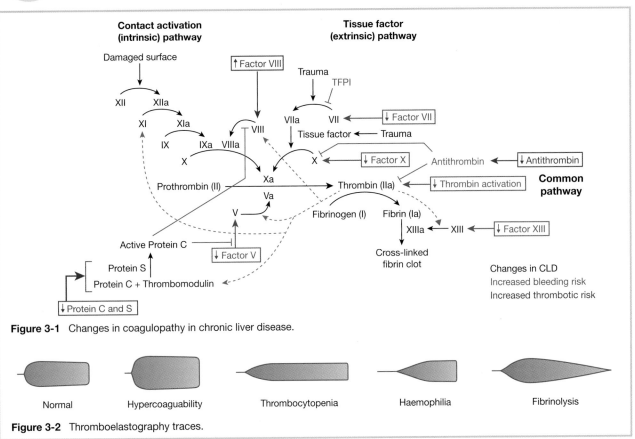

Figure 3-1 Changes in coagulopathy in chronic liver disease.

Figure 3-2 Thromboelastography traces.

Normal   Hypercoaguability   Thrombocytopenia   Haemophilia   Fibrinolysis

Hepatology at a Glance, First Edition. Deepak Joshi, Geri Keane and Alison Brind.
© 2015 John Wiley & Sons, Ltd. Published 2015 by John Wiley & Sons, Ltd. Companion website: www.ataglanceseries.com/hepatology

Normal coagulation

The coagulation cascade is divided into intrinsic, extrinsic and common pathways.

- Coagulation is activated following injury which results in the activation of tissue factor (TF) on the surface of injured cells.
- TF binds and activates factor VII, which activates factor X to Xa and IX to IXa.
- Factor IXa binds with VIIIa, which potentiates the activation of X to Xa further.
- Platelets are recruited to the site of injury and help accelerate the process by providing phospholipid membrane surface.
- Factor Xa induces the production of thrombin. Thrombin (IIa) is a key mediator of haemostasis and via a positive feedback loop it promotes further factor Xa activation.
- Thrombin converts fibrinogen into fibrin, potentiates platelet aggregation and activates factor XIII to XIIIa.
- Fibrin is a 'glue-like' substance that is the end product of the coagulation cascade.

Fibrinolysis

- Tissue plasminogen activator (TPA) is released from damaged or activated cells which activates plasminogen.
- Plasminogen is converted into plasmin which digests fibrin (or fibrinogen) into fibrinogen degradation products (FDPs).

Inhibitory factors

- Antithrombin inactivates factor Xa and thrombin.
- Proteins C and S (both vitamin-K-dependent proteins) are both synthesised in the liver. Both inactivate factors Va and VIIIa and therefore inhibit coagulation.
- Thrombomodulin activates protein C.
- Protein C inactivates TPA and therefore enhances fibrinolysis.
- Decreased factor V. Factor V Leiden occurs when the Leiden variant of factor V cannot be inactivated by activated protein C.
- Plasmin is inactivated by plasma α2-antiplasmin and α2-macroglobulin, both of which are synthesised in the liver.

Coagulopathy in liver disease

Historically, patients with coagulopathy in liver disease (CLD) are regarded to be at an increased risk of bleeding. More recently, a paradigm shift has occurred resulting in the recognition that there is also an increased risk of thrombosis, especially venous thrombosis. This can therefore make the management of patients with CLD extremely difficult with regards to bleeding risk versus anticoagulation. Therefore, the concept of 'auto-anticoagulation' does not exist. Changes in coagulopathy are shown in Figure 3.1. Coagulopathy of CLD can be similar to disseminated intravascular coagulation (DIC).

Increased bleeding risk

- Decreased non-endothelial cell-derived coagulation factors (II, V, VII, IX, X, XI and XIII);
- Decreased absorption of vitamin K resulting in decreased production in vitamin-K-dependent clotting factors (II, VII, IX and X) in jaundiced patients;
- Thrombocytopenia secondary to hypersplenism (portal hypertension) and abnormal platelet aggregation and function.
- Abnormalities of fibrinogen;
- Decreased thrombin activation.

Increased thrombotic risk

- Decreased proteins C and S;
- Decreased antithrombin levels;
- Decreased plasminogen;
- Increased endothelial cell-derived factor VIII;
- Increased von Willebrand factor (vWF);
- Decreased α2-antiplasmin and α2-macroglobulin.

Abnormal coagulation tests in CLD

Table 3.1

Test	Correction
↑ PT (10–14 s)	Fresh frozen plasma–prothrombin complex
↑ INR (>1.4)	Fresh frozen plasma–prothrombin complex
↑ APTT (30–40 s)	NA
↓ Fibrinogen	Cryoprecipitate
↓ Platelets ($<50 \times 10^9$/L)	Platelet transfusion
↓ Proteins C and S	NA
↓ Factor V	NA

Thromboelastography

Thromboelastography (TEG) is a specialised form of coagulation monitoring that uses viscoelastic coagulation tests. It is used routinely during cardiac surgery and there is increasing use during liver transplantation. A TEG trace is able to generate data regarding platelet function, fibrinogen levels, interaction between platelets and the coagulation system. It is a good test for fibrinolysis.

Approach to bleeding risk

- Review bleeding history.
- Review INR (may need correction if actively bleeding or having an invasive procedure).
- Platelets $>50\,000 \times 10^9$/L (if having an invasive procedure).
- Measure fibrinogen and support with cryoprecipitate.
- Assess for infection and treat accordingly.
- Control uraemia.
- Keep circulating volumes low.

4 Liver fibrosis

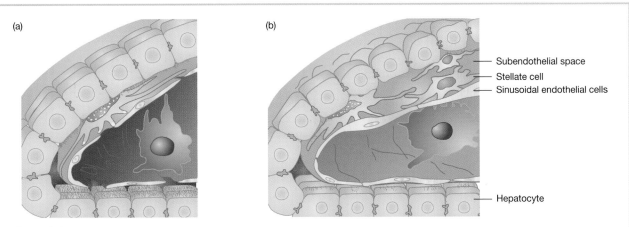

Subendothelial space
Stellate cell
Sinusoidal endothelial cells

Hepatocyte

Figure 4-1

(a) Normal liver. In this drawing of a normal sinsuoid, an hepatic stellate cell is depicted within the subendothelial space between hepatocytes and sinusoidal endothelial cells, where it extends foot processes encircling the sinusoid. The cells normally store retinoids within perinuclear lipid droplets (white circles) as shown. Microvilli depicted on hepatocytes indicate differentiated function, and sinusoidal endothelial cell fenestrae contribute to the rapid transport of solutes across the subendothelial space.

(b) Injured liver with fibrosis. This drawing shows an activated stellate cell with surrounding fibrillar matrix and loss of hepatocyte microvilli. In addition, sinusoidal porosity is reduced (i.e. loss of fenestrations, or pores).

Source: *Friedman SL (2004) Reproduced with permission of Nature Publishing Group.*

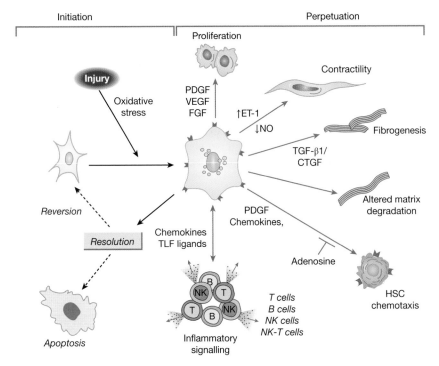

Figure 4-2 Initiation and perpetuation of hepatic stellate cells (HSCs).

Source: *Friedman SL (2008) Reproduced with permission of Elsevier.*

Hepatology at a Glance, First Edition. Deepak Joshi, Geri Keane and Alison Brind.
© 2015 John Wiley & Sons, Ltd. Published 2015 by John Wiley & Sons, Ltd. Companion website: www.ataglanceseries.com/hepatology

Liver fibrosis

Fibrosis or excessive accumulation of scar tissue occurs in response to any hepatocellular injury. It occurs in all patients with chronic liver injury but at variable rates depending on the underlying cause. In its early stages fibrosis is reversible but if the cause of the liver injury remains then progressive accumulation results in cirrhosis and the complications of end-stage liver disease. Fibrosis occurs in areas where injury is most severe.

Progression of fibrosis is usually non-linear and occurs over several years due to the liver's immense regenerative capacity and, at least in the early stages, to a balanced degradation and remodelling of fibrotic tissue. However, rapid fibrosis over months or even weeks has been described in patients with recurrent hepatitis C virus (HCV) infection post-liver transplantation and in patients with veno-occlusive disease.

Mechanisms of hepatic fibrosis

Normal liver

Type IV collagen, glycoproteins (fibronectin and laminin) and proteoglycans create a connective tissue matrix which forms the basement membrane in the space of Disse. Quiescent hepatic stellate cells (HSCs) reside in the space of Disse. It separates hepatocytes from the sinusoid epithelium in addition to providing support. There is a constant exchange of metabolites and solutes between blood and hepatocytes. The extracellular matrix (ECM) provides the 'scaffolding' for normal liver tissue. It consists of mainly of high-density fibrillar type 1 and III collagen (distributed according to a topographically defined architectural structure), collagen type IV, glycosaminoglycans, proteoglycans, fibronectin and hyaluronic acid (forming a basal membrane-like gel lining).

Liver injury

Hepatic fibrosis is a dynamic process. Liver injury results in increased secretion, decreased degradation and accumulation of the ECM. In addition there is a down-regulation of ECM-removing matrix metalloproteinases (MMPs) and an increase in tissue inhibitors of MMPs (TIMMPs). The composition of the ECM changes from a low-density matrix to a high-density matrix. The collagen content increases up to 10-fold, predominantly type I and III fibrillar collagens. The effectors of these changes are activated myofibroblasts deriving in large part from the activation of HSCs.

Activation of HSCs and other myofibroblasts is, in general, part of a chronic wound healing reaction and is associated with a phenotypical modulation of other liver non-parenchymal cells such as sinusoidal endothelial cells with loss of their typical fenestrations. This, together with the accumulation of fibrillar ECM in the space of Disse, results in reduced metabolite and oxygen exchange between hepatocytes and blood resulting in hepatocyte dysfunction and tissue hypoxia. The liver responds by increased angiogenesis, sinusoidal remodelling and HSC amplification. Increased contractility of HSCs leads to increased sinusoidal resistance and contributes to the genesis of portal hypertension. Progressive fibrosis results in disruption of the normal liver acinar architecture. Once the cause of liver injury is removed, HSCs revert to their quiescent state and are destroyed through apoptosis.

Hepatic stellate cells

HSCs are the main fibrogenic cell type in all forms of liver injury. In normal liver they contain vitamin A and store >60% of the body stores. HSC activation consists of two phases:
1 *Initiation:* HSCs become more responsive to stimuli.
2 *Perpetuation:* HSCs remain activated and generate fibrosis.

Activation of HSCs is the common pathway leading to hepatic fibrosis. It is accompanied by the loss of perinuclear retinoid droplets and change into a proliferative and contractile myofibroblast. HSCs are activated by a variety of pathways including necrosis, angiogenesis, steatosis and apoptosis. In addition, activated HSCs secrete chemokines and attract monocytes and lymphocytes, thus leading to the amplification of the fibro-inflammatory process.

HSCs proliferate rapidly and migrate to the site of injury in response to a variety of chemokines and cytokines including platelet derived growth factor β (PDGF-β), vascular endothelial growth factor (VEGF) and insulin-like growth factor 1 (IGF-1). Transforming growth factor β1 (TGF-β1) is the most potent fibogenic cytokine and is produced by HSCs, sinusoidal endothelial cells and Kupffer cells. TGF-β is a potent stimulator of collagen I production.

Up-regulation of fibrogenic pathways

Activation of HSCs results in the secretion of pro-inflammatory chemokines and cytokines (e.g. IL-6, NF-κB, TNF-α). A positive feedback loop is created in which inflammatory cells and fibrogenic cells stimulate each other and amplify fibrosis. Fibrosis is potentiated further by production of reactive oxidative species (ROS), angiogenic cytokines (VEGF, PDGF) and bacterial lipopolysaccharide (LPS) via bacterial translocation from the gut.

Risk factors

Oestrogens appear to be protective, with slower fibrosis rates noted amongst women than men. Single nuclear polymorphisms in a variety of genes have been identified that confer an increased risk of developing fibrosis (e.g. Toll-like receptor 4 (TLR4), complement C5).

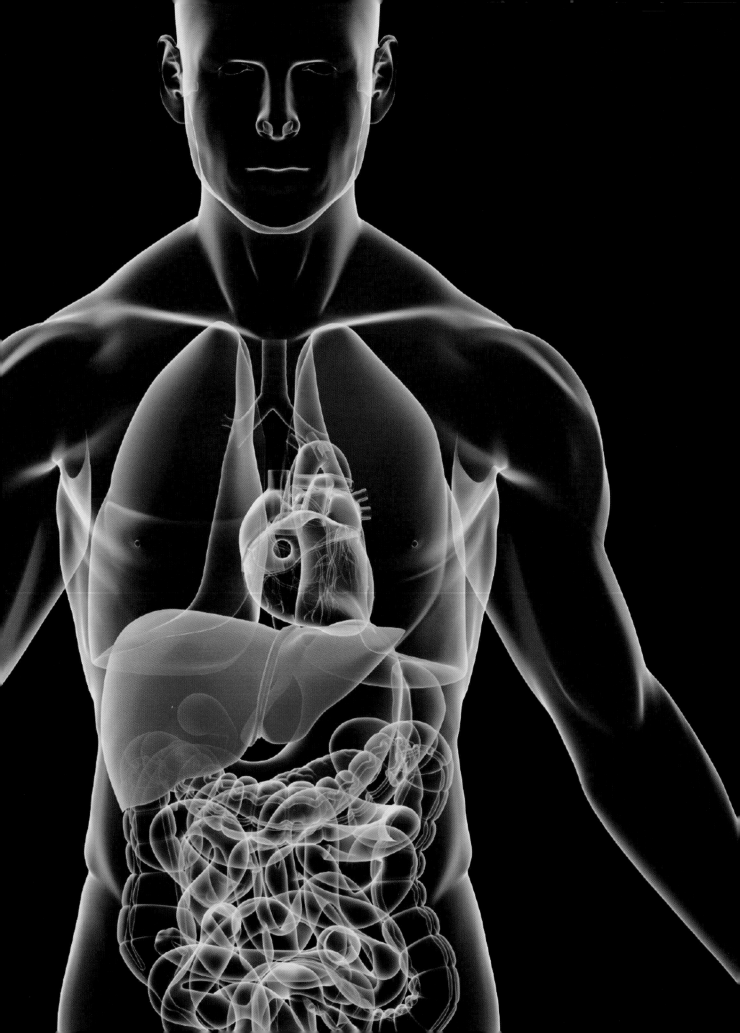

Evaluation of liver disease

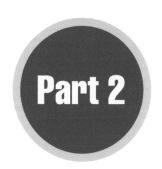

Part 2

Chapters

Visit the companion website at
www.ataglanceseries.com/hepatology
to test yourself on these topics

5 Clinical history

New patients

Presenting complaint:
What has brought you to hospital/clinic today?
(NB: Some patients will be asymptomatic and attending outpatients because their LFTs were found to be abnormal on routine testing)

Past medical history:
Do you have any other medical problems?
Have you ever had any operations?
(The GP referral letter often contains a list of medical problems for reference)

Drug history:
Do you have any drug allergies?
What medicines are you taking?
Do you take any other vitamins or supplements?

History of presenting complaint:
How long have you had [the presenting symptom]?
Is it there all the time or does it come and go?
Have you noticed any other problems such as yellowing of your eyes/skin (jaundice), itching, bruising, loss of appetite, weight loss?
(NB: Accompanying family members may be able to provide further information)

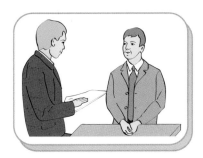

Family history:
Are there any medical problems that run in the family?
Has anyone ever had liver disease or liver cancer?

Risk factors for acquired liver disease:
• Excess alcohol consumption
• Obesity/metabolic syndrome
• Illicit drugs
• Travel
• Tattoos/body piercings
• Blood transfusion
• High risk sexual activity
• Job (e.g. healthcare worker)
• Pregnancy

Systematic review:
Taking each system in turn, enquire about multisystemic features of liver disease?
• *Neurology:* Abnormal movements, i.e. chorea, memory impairment or peripheral neuropathy
• *Cardiovascular:* Heart failure
• *Respiratory:* Emphysema
• *Gastrointestinal:* Inflammatory bowel disease, coeliac's disease, chronic pancreatitis
• *Endocrine:* Diabetes, obesity, thyroid disease
• *Rheumatology/Dermatology:* Swollen joints, changes in skin pigmentation or rashes, sicca syndrome

All patients with chronic liver disease:

Evidence of decompensation:
• Hepatic encephalopathy/confusion
• Jaundice
• Ascites
• Gastrointestinal bleeding/coagulopathy

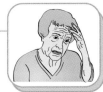

Surveillance:
• Varices (see Chapter 14)
• Hepatocellular carcinoma (see Chapter 40)
• Nutritional status – particularly in ALD (see Chapter 49)
• Osteopenia or osteoporosis – particularly in patients with ALD, autoimmune or cholestatic liver disease (see Chapters 31–34)

Hepatology at a Glance, First Edition. Deepak Joshi, Geri Keane and Alison Brind.
© 2015 John Wiley & Sons, Ltd. Published 2015 by John Wiley & Sons, Ltd. Companion website: www.ataglanceseries.com/hepatology

A thorough history is fundamental to determining the final diagnosis in liver disease. The clinical history should focus on symptoms: their onset, duration, associations and related risk factors. Remember that some patients will be asymptomatic and attending outpatients because their liver biochemistry was found to be abnormal on routine testing.

Common presenting complaints

Jaundice: This is by far the most obvious symptom of liver disease. In adults it is commonly caused by biliary obstruction (due to malignancy or choledocholithiasis), acute hepatitis, decompensated chronic liver disease, alcoholic hepatitis or drug-induced liver disease. Chronic mild jaundice may be seen in Gilbert's syndrome, compensated chronic liver disease or haemolysis.

Decompensation: The development of new onset (or progression of existing) jaundice, ascites, encephalopathy, coagulopathy or variceal bleeding/anaemia in the context of existing chronic liver disease. It can also be indicative of the development of HCC. It requires specific management (see Chapters 14–16 and 19).

Anorexia: Anorexia and weight loss are common symptoms of malignancy but can occur in chronic liver disease of any severity.

Abdominal pain: Rare in parenchymal liver disease but a common feature of cholecystitis and choledocholithiasis.

Fatigue and pruritus: Non-specific symptoms that are particularly prevalent in cholestatic liver disease.

Fever: Fever is a common feature of infection (e.g. viral hepatitis, liver abscesses or ascending cholangitis, e.g. Charcot's triad: fever, pain and jaundice).

Dark urine and pale stools: Features of extrahepatic biliary obstruction.

History of presenting complaint

If symptoms are present enquire about their onset, duration, precipitating or relieving factors and any associated features.

Risk factors for primary liver disease (+ social history)

Most liver diseases are more prevalent in certain populations and/or are associated with established risk factors. If the underlying aetiology is unclear, screening for risk factors can be helpful in determining the cause of the underlying liver disease. Risk factors often overlap with a traditional social history, so commonly clinicians incorporate both parts of the clinical history at this point.

Suspected viral hepatitis

• *Hepatitis A/E:* exposure to a possible oro-faecal transmission source (e.g. recent travel to an endemic area or residence or work in an institution, e.g. prison or pre-school).

• *Hepatitis B/C:* country of birth (e.g. high national prevalence of viral hepatitis increases likelihood of materno-fetal transmission), acquired blood-borne virus risk (e.g. IV drug use, tattoos, body piercing), high-risk sexual activity, partner with hepatitis, occupation (e.g. health care workers), blood transfusion (before 1991 in the UK or abroad at any time).

• Document previous hepatitis immunisations, if known.

Suspected alcoholic liver disease (ALD): Document current and historical alcohol consumption. Collateral from family may also be useful. Smoking status.

Suspected non-alcoholic steatohepatitis (NASH): Ask about risk factors for metabolic syndrome (e.g. diabetes or hypertension).

Toxins: Document current occupation and any potential occupational exposure to hepatotoxins.

Past medical history

Current and past medical problems in chronological order. For patients with chronic liver disease include previous episodes of decompensation.

Drug history

Include allergies, currently prescribed medications, over-the-counter (OTC) medications, herbs and supplements. If a drug-induced liver injury is likely, also ask about additional short courses of medications (e.g. antibiotics) and any medications that have been stopped recently. In all patients with acute liver failure ask about recent paracetamol ingestion and the possibility of inadvertent or intentional overdose.

Family history

Rare inherited liver diseases such as haemochromatosis, Wilson's disease, α1-antitrypsin deficiency, cystic fibrosis and glycogen storage diseases can present *de novo* but more commonly run within families. If one of these conditions is suspected ask about other affected family members and keep in mind others who may be at risk or require screening.

Systematic review

The systematic review should determine if there are any multisystemic features or complications associated with the underlying liver disease.

• *Neurological disease:* chorea or altered behaviour (e.g. Wilson's disease) or peripheral neuropathy, Wernicke–Korsakoff syndrome, dementia (ALD);

• *Cardiac disease:* cardiomyopathy (ALD or haemachromatosis) or right-sided heart failure (congestive hepatopathy);

• *Respiratory disease:* emphysema (α1-antitrypsin deficiency);

• *Gastrointestinal disease:* inflammatory bowel disease, coeliac disease (primary sclerosing cholangitis or autoimmune hepatitis), chronic pancreatitis (ALD, haemochromatosis or cystic fibrosis);

• *Endocrine disease:* diabetes/metabolic syndrome (NASH);

• *Rheumatological/dermatological disease:* arthritis (autoimmune hepatitis, acute hepatitis B, haemochromatosis or sarcoidosis), osteopenia or osteoporosis (all chronic liver diseases), rash or changes in skin pigmentation (porphyria cutanea tarda and 'bronze diabetes' in haemochromatosis).

6 Liver examination

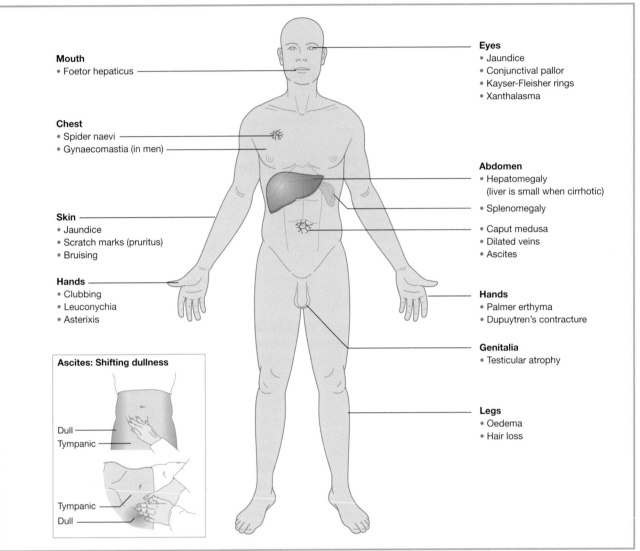

Mouth
- Foetor hepaticus

Chest
- Spider naevi
- Gynaecomastia (in men)

Skin
- Jaundice
- Scratch marks (pruritus)
- Bruising

Hands
- Clubbing
- Leuconychia
- Asterixis

Eyes
- Jaundice
- Conjunctival pallor
- Kayser-Fleisher rings
- Xanthalasma

Abdomen
- Hepatomegaly
  (liver is small when cirrhotic)
- Splenomegaly
- Caput medusa
- Dilated veins
- Ascites

Hands
- Palmer erthyma
- Dupuytren's contracture

Genitalia
- Testicular atrophy

Legs
- Oedema
- Hair loss

Ascites: Shifting dullness

Dull
Tympanic

Tympanic
Dull

Hepatology at a Glance, First Edition. Deepak Joshi, Geri Keane and Alison Brind.
© 2015 John Wiley & Sons, Ltd. Published 2015 by John Wiley & Sons, Ltd. Companion website: www.ataglanceseries.com/hepatology

The standard abdominal examination in liver disease is tailored to identify the aetiology of the underlying liver disease and to look for signs of decompensation.

Hands signs

Table 6.1

Sign	Cause
Leuconychia	Hypoalbuminaemia
Koilonychia	Iron deficiency anaemia, haemochromatosis
Clubbing	Chronic liver disease (e.g. cirrhosis or HCC), as well as many any non-hepatological causes
Dupuytren's contracture	Excess alcohol, familial
Palmar erythema	Chronic liver disease, thyrotoxicosis, pregnancy
Asterixis	Flapping tremor of the hands consistent with HE and decompensation
Fine tremor	Alcohol withdrawal

Skin and musculoskeletal signs

• Skin pigmentation: jaundice due to hyperbilirubinaemia becomes clinically detectable at 2–3 times the upper limit of normal. It is often associated with significant pruritus and skin excoriations. In the late stages of haemochromatosis, iron deposition in the skin can lead to a bronze skin pigmentation.
• Rashes (e.g. porphyria cutanea tarda) on the dorsum of the hands is associated with haemochromatosis or HCV.
• Bruising and petechiae are suggestive of a prolonged clotting time or thrombocytopenia.
• Needle tract marks are indicative of illicit drug use.
• Proximal muscle wasting is a common feature of advanced liver disease.

Facial signs

• Eye signs include yellowing of the sclera (jaundice), conjunctival pallor (anaemia), Kayser–Fleischer rings (a greenish-brown ring at edge of iris, best observed with a slit-lamp is indicative of Wilson's disease – Chapter 36), xanthalasma (yellow deposits around the eyes seen in primary biliary cirrhosis – Chapter 32).
• Facial signs include parotid enlargement with a 'moon face' or pseudo-Cushing's, commonly seen in alcoholic liver disease.

Chest signs

Gynaecomastia (palpable breast tissue in males), spider naevi (central arteriole feeding multiple draining capillaries, present on the face or upper chest wall) and loss of axillary hair are suggestive of chronic liver disease. More than five spider naevai in women and more than three in men are considered pathological. Finally palpate for cervical lymphadenopathy i.e. virchows node (tousier's sign).

Abdominal signs
Inspection
• Abdominal scars (e.g. subcostal, midline laparotomy);
• Abdominal mass (e.g. organomegaly or mass lesion);
• Dilated veins or caput medusa: portal hypertension;
• Ascites: confirmed clinically by presence of a fluid thrill or shifting dullness (see examination technique in figure).

Percussion and palpation
Enquire about abdominal pain and begin palpation or percussion away from the site of pain. Palpate all four quadrants superficially, then deeply. Next, assess for organomegaly.
Organomegaly: To examine for hepatomegaly ask the patient to take slow deep breaths and palpate in steps from the right lower quadrant towards the subcostal margin. An enlarged liver is defined as a liver edge that is palpable more than 2 cm below the right costal margin. In emphysema, the liver may be pushed down by the expanded lungs, giving the impression of hepatomegaly; however, correlation with liver span will reveal a normal-sized liver. Percussion from the nipple line to the level of the umbilicus determines liver span. A normal liver span in men is 10–12 cm and 8–11 cm in women. Cirrhotic livers are typically shrunken, fibrotic and no longer palpable. To assess for splenomegaly, start by palpating from the right iliac fossa towards the left subcostal margin. The spleen is usually palpable when it is double its normal size and is recognisable by its distinctive 'notch'. Percussion along the same line will confirm palpation findings.
Panceaticobiliary: Pain in the right upper quadrant that is aggravated by inspiration (Murphy's sign) is indicative of cholecystitis. A painless palpable gallbladder with jaundice is less likely to be associated with gallstone disease and more likely to be the result of a lesion in the head of the pancreas (Courvoisier's law). Jaundice without peripheral stigmata of chronic liver disease is more likely to be pancreatico-biliary in origin.
Kidneys: Ballot each kidney in turn. Polycystic kidneys are usually palpable and are associated with the development of liver cysts.
Ascites: A dull percussion note in the flanks in a patient with a distended abdomen is suggestive of ascites. Its presence can be confirmed clinically by looking for a fluid thrill or the presence of shifting dullness (see figure). If present assess for the presence of a hepatic hydrothorax (pleural effusion).

Auscultation
Auscultation over the liver occasionally demonstrates the following rare clinical signs:
• *Friction rub:* liver cancer, Fitz-Hugh–Curtis syndrome, liver infarct or following a liver biopsy;
• *Venous hum:* portal hypertension or Cruveilhier–Baumgarten syndrome;
• *Arterial systolic bruit:* liver cancer, acute alcoholic hepatitis or arteriovenous malformation.

Signs of decompensation
• Encephalopathy and altered mental state;
• Asterixis (coarse flapping tremor of the hands);
• Fetor hepaticus (sweet musty odour): occurs in late-stage liver disease;
• Bruising suggesting coagulopathy;
• Jaundice;
• Evidence of gastrointestinal haemorrhage (per rectum examination).

7 Liver function tests

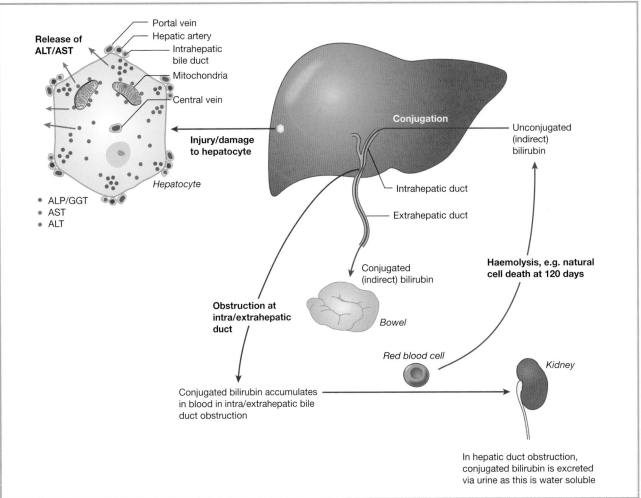

Definition

Liver function tests (LFTs) are routinely measured in blood. They reflect the synthetic function and evidence of liver cell damage. LFTs are frequently performed in clinical practice to investigate symptoms, signs suggesting liver disease, evidence of liver damage in individuals at risk of liver disease (e.g. heavy alcohol drinkers) and to monitor effects of treatment.

Box 7.1 Factors to consider when interpreting LFTs

- Clinical context
- Dynamic nature of changes: acute/chronic
- Pattern of derangement
- Degree of derangement

Patterns of abnormal LFTs

- *Hepatocellular:* raised alanine transaminase (ALT), aspartate transaminase (AST);
- *Cholestatic:* raised alkaline phosphatase (ALP) and gamma-glutamyltransferase (GGT);
- *Mixed:* raised ALT/AST and ALP/GGT together.

Markers of synthetic function

Bilirubin synthesis and metabolism

Bilirubin is produced by the reticuloendothelial system (spleen, liver and bone marrow) predominately from the breakdown of haem. Unconjugated bilirubin is bound to albumin and taken up into hepatocytes. It is then cleaved from albumin before being conjugated to glucuronic acid in the endoplasmic reticulum (UGT). Conjugated bilirubin is then excreted across the canalicular membrane into the bile canaliculus via an ATP-dependent pump. In the small bowel, bacteria deconjugates bilirubin to produce urobilinogen. Ninety per cent of urobilinogen is broken down into urobilin and stercobilin (brown coloured), which is excreted into faeces. Ten per cent of urobilinogen is reabsorbed into the portal vein, some of which re-enters the liver via the enterohepatic circulation while most bypasses the liver and is excreted by the kidneys.

Albumin

The half-life of albumin is approximately 21 days, with a degradation rate of approximately 4% per day. It is reduced in subacute and chronic parenchymal liver disease (e.g. cirrhosis). Interpretation can be difficult as albumin can also be reduced in malnutrition, nephrotic syndrome, protein losing enteropathy, sepsis and acute inflammatory illnesses.

PT and INR

PT and INR are the most sensitive markers of liver function. PT half-life is just under 3 days. It is dependent on hepatic synthesis of clotting factors (see Chapter 4). Reduced PT and therefore increased PT time and INR are seen in acute and chronic parenchymal liver disease in relation to severity. The PT and INR are raised in cases of vitamin K malabsorption (e.g. cholestasis).

Ammonia

See Chapter 19.

Markers of liver damage

Alanine transaminase

Highly specific for hepatocyte damage. Plasma half-life of approximately 36–48 hours.

Aspartate transaminase

Released by hepatocytes after damage. Plasma half-life of 12–24 hours.

Also released from skeletal muscle, cardiac muscle and red blood cells. AST : ALT ratio >1 indicates more significant liver damage than ALT rise alone.

Alkaline phosphatase

Secreted by apical border of hepatocytes and cholangiocytes. Also secreted by placenta, ileal mucosa, kidney and bone. Plasma half-life of 72 hours. If elevated then ALP isoenzymes can be used to differentiate the source. Significant elevations are mainly seen in diseases associated with either intra-or extrahepatic cholestasis, but smaller elevations of the enzyme (2–3 times the upper limits of normal) can be seen in all types of liver disorders. Can also be induced by drugs (e.g. anticonvulsants).

Gamma-glutamyltransferase

Serum activity is primarily from liver cholangiocytes. A membrane-bound enzyme found in proximal renal tubule, pancreas and small intestine. Plasma half-life of 7–10 days. GGT is more sensitive than ALP in obstructive liver disease but can also be raised in:

- Alcohol ingestion;
- Non-alcoholic fatty liver disease (NAFLD);
- Diabetes, hyperthyroidism, rheumatoid arthritis, chronic obstructive pulmonary disease (COPD); and
- Drugs (e.g. anticonvulsants).

8 Radiology in liver disease

Indication for imaging	Imaging features	
Abnormal LFTs Jaundice Abdominal pain, HCC surveillance	Ultrasound with Doppler is an excellent first line screening investigation HCC surveillance: 6-monthly US is recommended for cirrhotic patients (Child-Pugh stage A, B and stage C if awaiting liver transplantation), non-cirrhotic HBV carriers with active hepatitis or a family history of HCC and patients with chronic HCV and advanced liver fibrosis	
Benign liver mass e.g. simple cyst	If typical radiological features of benign disease are present no further imaging or follow-up is typically required	
Indeterminate liver mass	Nodules greater than 2 cm that demonstrate 'venous washout' are diagnostic of HCC and histological confirmation prior to treatment is not mandatory Small indeterminate liver lesions are a common finding on CT and US. If clinical uncertainty remains following CT, tumour markers, complementary imaging (e.g. MRI), liver biopsy or short-interval follow-up imaging (at 3 months) can be used to clarify aetiology. Nodules less than 2 cm are best characterised by MRI	
Malignant liver mass	All lesions with typical features of malignant disease should be fully staged with a chest, abdomen and pelvis CT to exclude extrahepatic disease. Complementary imaging with MR (see text) or PET/CT may better delineate tumour extent as well as biliary and vascular anatomy prior to intervention	
Cholangiopathies	A liver US is a very sensitive test for detecting gallbladder stones and intrahepatic biliary dilation. The extrahepatic biliary tree is frequently obscured and if distal biliary obstruction is suspected an MRCP or contrast enhanced CT is recommended to guide therapy (see text). In cholangiocarcinoma, MRCP is recommended in addition to CT to delineate biliary anatomy	
Interventional Radiology	CT angiography is used to deliver transarterial embolisation and trans-arterial chemoembolisation and to determine the site of bleeding in suspected liver haemorrhage. In these situations interventional radiologists can often embolise feeding vessels preventing the need for major liver surgery. Interventional radiology can also facilitate transjugular biopsies and the insertion of shunts such as Transjugular Intrahepatic Portosystemic Shunts (TIPS)	

Ultrasound

Ultrasound (US) images are formed from high frequency sound waves that are reflected to differing degrees by the underlying tissues.

Indications:
- Jaundice and/or abnormal LFTs;
- Abdominal, flank, back pain or referred pain;
- Further assessment of abdominal mass or organomegaly;

Hepatology at a Glance, First Edition. Deepak Joshi, Geri Keane and Alison Brind.
© 2015 John Wiley & Sons, Ltd. Published 2015 by John Wiley & Sons, Ltd. Companion website: www.ataglanceseries.com/hepatology

- Screening and surveillance (e.g. HCC);
- Abdominal trauma (e.g. FAST scan);
- In planning or guiding invasive procedures (e.g. liver biopsy);
- Assessment of liver vasculature (e.g. colour Doppler US) can detect portal vein thrombosis or Budd–Chiari syndrome;
- Clarification of other imaging findings (e.g. US) can detect >90% of gallstones, which are rarely seen on CT unless calcified. US can also differentiate between solid and cystic lesions effectively when localisation is feasible. IV contrast (microbubble agents) or Doppler can further improve sensitivity.

Advantages: Simple, cheap, widely available, non-invasive, with no ionising radiation dose and can be performed at the bedside.

Disadvantages: Operator dependent, views may be obscured in obese patients or by overlying bowel gas. If steatosis or cirrhosis is present the sensitivity for detecting liver lesions or tumours is further reduced. If there is a high index of clinical suspicion of HCC and the US is normal, then cross-sectional imaging (CT or MRI) is recommended.

Computed tomography scan

Three-dimensional CT images are formed from continuous spiral scanning using multiple X-ray tubes and detectors. IV contrast enhances vascular structures and liver parenchyma and improves the detection of focal liver lesions.

Indications:
- Further characterisation of known liver lesions;
- Staging of malignancy;
- Assessment of liver trauma (often in combination with CT angiography);
- Assessment of pancreatico-biliary disease. CT is the gold standard investigation for diagnosing pancreatic pathology;
- In planning or guiding invasive procedures (e.g. liver biopsy).

Advantages: Readily available, very short scanning time, excellent visualisation of all abdominal organs.

Disadvantages: Associated ionising radiation dose (8 mSv – equivalent to 400 chest X-rays), contrast nephropathy can occur particularly in those with pre-existing renal disease. Contraindicated in pregnancy.

Magnetic resonance imaging

Magnetic resonance (MR) images are formed from the radiofrequency signal obtained from relaxation of tissue protons (water) following a radiofrequency pulse applied within a strong magnetic field.

Indications:
- Further characterisation of parenchymal pathology and focal liver masses;
- MR cholangiopancreatography (MRCP) is the diagnostic test of choice for evaluating the bile ducts (e.g. detecting intraluminal stones or stricturing disease).

Advantages: No ionising radiation dose.

Disadvantages: Lengthy scanning time. Contraindications to MR include metal implants (especially pacemakers and aneurysm clips), claustrophobia, morbid obesity, and pregnancy (first trimester).

Advanced endoscopy
Endoscopic retrograde cholangiopancreatography

Endoscopic retrograde cholangiopancreatography (ERCP) enables fluoroscopic and increasingly direct visualisation of the biliary tree and/or pancreatic duct. ERCP is primarily undertaken for therapeutic intervention (e.g. stone removal, stent insertion or to obtain pathological specimens). It is associated with a morbidity of 3–5% (gastrointestinal bleeding, perforation, pancreatitis).

Endoscopic ultrasound

Echoendoscopes incorporate a US probe into the tip of the endoscope. Endoscopic US (EUS) provides high-quality US images of structures in the wall and adjacent to the wall of the stomach and duodenum such as the pancreas, bile duct and gallbladder. It can accurately define pancreatico-biliary tumour margins preoperatively as well as providing pathological specimens for histological confirmation.

Interventional radiology
Percutaneous transhepatic cholangiopancreatography

Fluoroscopic assessment of the biliary tree can be performed endoscopically or percutaneously. In most centres, the endoscopic approach is used first line. In complex strictures a combined percutaneous and endoscopic approach is sometimes used. A dilated intrahepatic biliary tree is normally required for percutaneous access.

Hepatic angiography

CT angiography depicts the branching pattern and patency of hepatic vessels. Images are equivalent to catheter angiography and CT liver imaging can be displayed simultaneously.

Indications: Assessment of bleeding post-liver biopsy, liver trauma with suspected vascular injury, arteriovenous malformations or haemobilia, or for tumour chemoembolisation. At many institutions, CT angiography has become the method of choice for evaluating living related liver donors and recipients prior to transplantation, as liver parenchyma, volumes and vasculature can be evaluated simultaneously.

Nuclear medicine
Positron emission tomography

Positron emission tomography (PET) is a functional imaging technique that detects an increased metabolic rate, which is common in most tumours. (18 F) 2-fluoro-2-deoxy-D-glucose (FDG) is the most commonly used tracer. PET is commonly combined with CT so anatomical and functional information can be gained simultaneously.

Indication: Assessment of liver lesions that are suspected to be malignant.

Disadvantages: Infection and inflammation can give similar images so differentiation may be challenging. Not widely available and expensive.

Cholescintigraphy

Hepatobiliary iminodiacetic acid (HIDA) scan is used to assess gallbladder function. A radioactive tracer is injected intravenously which is subsequently excreted by the biliary system. A normal gallbladder is visualised within 1 hour. No visualisation within 4 hours is indicative of either cholecystitis or cystic duct obstruction.

Indication: To provide functional information in pre- and postoperative patients with known or suspected hepatobiliary disease.

Disadvantages: Invasive, costly and time-consuming test.

9 Liver biopsy

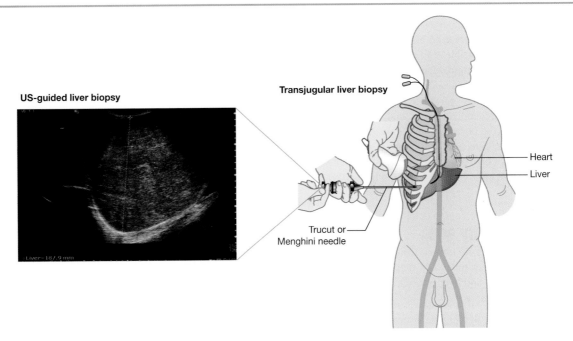

Table 9-1 Histological assessment of liver fibrosis.

Appearance	Metavir grade	Ishak stage	Histological findings
Portal area Central area Hepatocytes Lobule	F0	0	Normal liver
Fibrous portal expansion	F1	1	Fibrous expansion of some of the portal areas
Bridging fibrosis	F2	2–3	Fibrous expansion of most portal areas. Ishak stage 3 is differentiated by the presence of occasional portal-to-portal bridging fibrosis
	F3	4–5	Fibrous expansion of portal areas with marked portal-to-portal and portal-to-central bridging fibrosis. If occasional nodules are present this is indicative of Ishak stage 5
	F4	6	Cirrhosis

Hepatology at a Glance, First Edition. Deepak Joshi, Geri Keane and Alison Brind.
© 2015 John Wiley & Sons, Ltd. Published 2015 by John Wiley & Sons, Ltd. Companion website: www.ataglanceseries.com/hepatology

Indications

A liver biopsy was first used to determine the aetiology of chronic liver disease more than 130 years ago and remains the most common indication for the test. A liver biopsy can also be used to determine the stage and severity of liver disease. In NAFLD, it is useful in determining the degree of fibrosis and excluding other causes of abnormal liver biochemistry. In alcohol-related liver disease, it can differentiate alcoholic hepatitis from decompensated cirrhosis, which often present similarly. In chronic viral hepatitis, aminotransferases are unreliable markers of fibrosis and a liver biopsy is frequently used to determine the presence of significant fibrosis and to guide antiviral treatment.

In autoimmune hepatitis, serial biopsies every few years are used to guide treatment, predict disease progression and overall prognosis. In metabolic liver diseases such as haemachomatosis and Wilson's disease, a liver biopsy can be used to measure iron and copper levels within the liver parenchyma. A liver biopsy can also be cultured or examined for acid-fast bacilli (AFBs) to diagnose infections such as tuberculosis (TB). Post-transplantation liver biopsies are used to assess for graft rejection (humoral, acute, chronic), infections (e.g. cytomegalovirus), bile duct obstruction, hepatic artery and/or portal vein thrombosis, drug toxicity, recurrent disease or neoplastic disease.

However, the need for a liver biopsy in certain situations remains controversial. For example, in patients with intrahepatic cholestasis, persistently elevated E_2-antimitochondrial antibody (AMA) and raised immunoglobulin M (IgM) levels are diagnostic of primary biliary cirrhosis (PBC) and a biopsy is rarely necessary. In primary sclerosing cholangitis (PSC), imaging is often of greater diagnostic utility as histological features are not unique. In malignant disease, there is a small risk of tumour seeding so only tumours that remain indeterminate following imaging or unresectable are recommended for sampling (see Chapter 40).

In the future, non-invasive serum markers may replace some current indications for liver biopsy (see Chapter 10).

Types of liver biopsy

• Percutaneous liver biopsy (see Table 9.1; e.g transthoracic or subcostal). Undertaken with US guidance.
• Transjugular liver biopsies (see Table 9.1) are performed with fluoroscopic guidance and cardiac monitoring. The catheter is passed through the internal jugular vein, right atrium, inferior vena cava (IVC) and into the hepatic veins. The biopsy needle is then advanced 1–2 cm to the liver to obtain the biopsy. Gentle suction keeps the biopsy within the needle as the catheter is withdrawn. The transfemoral approach is an alternative.
• Intraoperative liver biopsy: open or laparoscopic.
• Endoscopic: EUS can be used to biopsy the liver parenchyma (although rarely performed).

Complications

Many patients experience mild right upper quadrant pain for a few days following the procedure but this is generally well controlled with simple analgesia. Morbidity is 1–5% (e.g. bleeding, subcapsular haematoma or pneumothorax). Mortality is 1 in 1000–10 000

cases, therefore a clear indication for the test is mandated. Patients are typically recovered in the right lateral position and monitored for at least 6 hours before discharge.

Contraindications

• Uncooperative patient;
• Extrahepatic biliary obstruction, due to risk of bile leak;
• Abnormal clotting: INR >1.3 and platelets <50 mm³;
• Ascites: increased risk of bleeding and failed procedure;
• Cystic lesions: imaging is a better diagnostic entity and there is a small risk of precipitating abdominal dissemination of hydatid disease;
• Amyloidosis: increased risk of bleeding.

Adequacy of specimen

Although a liver biopsy remains the gold standard test for the assessment of fibrosis, the average liver biopsy consists of 1/50 000 of the total hepatic mass and hence sampling error may miss the diagnosis of cirrhosis in up to one-third of patients. It is generally recognised that the larger and less traumatised the specimen, the more accurate the histological assessment. However, specimen adequacy has to be balanced against feasibility and clinical safety. Although there are no universally agreed guidelines, a sample of at least 1.5 cm in length, with at least 6–8 complete portal tracts is recommended.

Staining

Pathology stains vary among centres. The minimum recommended is a haematoxylin and eosin (H&E) and a reliable method for connective tissue staining (e.g. reticulin, trichrome, Sirius Red). Other recommended routine stains include the periodic acid–Schiff (PAS) after diastase digestion as screening procedure for α1-antitrypsin deficiency, a stain for copper-associated protein, elastic fibres and hepatitis B surface antigen (e.g. orcein, Victoria blue) and a Perls' stain for iron. Further stains that can be considered as required for particular purposes include rubeanic acid (copper in Wilson's disease), AFB (TB), Congo red (amyloid), cytokeratins 7 or 19 (for assessment of bile duct loss) or ubiquitin for Mallory bodies (alcoholic liver disease). Biopsies may also be sent to specialist centres to perform the following techniques where indicated: electron microscopy for investigation of metabolic/storage disease or *in situ* hybridisation (e.g. in Epstein–Barr virus).

Interpretation of a liver biopsy

The pathologist begins by making an overall assessment of the liver architecture and severity of inflammation and fibrosis, recorded by grade or stage (see scoring systems in Table 9.1). A detailed morphological description of the specimen is then made, highlighting any architectural abnormalities within the portal tracts, parenchyma and the outcome of any special stains performed including negative results. A final diagnosis or differential is then suggested. Of note, many pathological features in liver disease overlap, therefore clinical context is essential for accurate interpretation.

10 Non-invasive markers of fibrosis

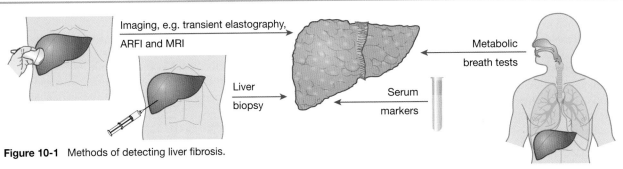

Figure 10-1 Methods of detecting liver fibrosis.

Table 10-1 Performance of different noninvasive serum scores to detect significant (≥F2) liver fibrosis and cirrhosis (F4) in patients with chronic viral hepatitis. Source: *Papastergiou et al. (2012).*

Method	Included serum markers	Etiology	Sensitivity (%) 2F2	Sensitivity (%) F4	Specificity (%) 2F2	Specificity (%) F4v
APRI	AST, platelets	HCV HBV	41–91 64.4–70.8	57–89 42.9	47–95 70.5–87	75–93 85.4
Fibrotest	γ-GT, haptoglobin, bilirubin, A1 apolipoprotein, α2-macroglobulin	HCV HBV	65–77 80.8	50–87 55.6	72–91 90	70–92.9 96.3
Forns Index	Age, γ-GT, cholesterol, platelets	HCV HBV	79.8–94 58.3	NA NA	61.2–95 78.3	NA NA
FIB-4	Age, ALT, AST, platelets	HCV/HIV HBV	37.6–74.3 71	NA NA	80.1–98.2 73	NA NA
Fibrometer	Platelets, prothrombin time, macroglobulin, AST, hyaluronate, age, urea	HCV HBV	80.5–89 NA	94.1 NA	84.1–89.9 NA	87.6 NA
Hepascore	Age, sex, α2-macroglobulin, hyaluronate, bilirubin, γ-GT	HCV	53.8–8.2	71–76.5	65–92	84–89.8
Enhanced liver fibrosis score (ELF)	N-terminal propeptide of collagen type III, hyaluronate, TIMP-1, age	HCV/HBV	90	NA	31	NA
Fibroindex	Platelet count, AST and γ-globulin	HCV	36	NA	97	NA
Fibrospect	α2-macroglobulin, hyaluronate and TIMP-1	HCV	71.8–93	NA	66–73.9	NA

Table 10-2 Indicative performance characteristics of non-invasive methods to assess advanced (F3-F4) liver fibrosis in patients with NAFLD/NASH. Source: *Papastergiou et al. (2012).*

Score	Serum markers/Fibroscan	Cut-off	Sensitivity (%)	Specificity (%)
FIB-4	Age, ALT, AST, platelets	1.3 2.67 3.25	74–85 34 26	65–71 98 98
NAFLD fibrosis score	Age, BMI, platelets, albumin, AST/ALT, IFG/diabetes	−1.455 0.676	78–82 33–51	58–77 98
BARD	BMI, AST/ALT, diabetes	2–4 2	NA 51–89	NA 44–77
ELF	N-terminal propeptide of collagen type III, hyaluronate, TIMP-1	−1.0281 0.2112	90 80	75 90
Fibrotest	α2-macroglobulin, apolipoprotein A1, haptoglobin, bilirubin, γ-GT	0.30 0.70	92 25	71 97
Fibrometer	Platelets, prothrombin time, macroglobulin, AST, hyaluronate, age, urea	NA	79	96

Hepatology at a Glance, First Edition. Deepak Joshi, Geri Keane and Alison Brind.
© 2015 John Wiley & Sons, Ltd. Published 2015 by John Wiley & Sons, Ltd. Companion website: www.ataglanceseries.com/hepatology

In all patients with chronic liver disease, staging of liver fibrosis is an important predictor of prognosis and is essential to guide management. Until recently a liver biopsy has been the only method for diagnosing and assessing liver fibrosis. However, it has a number of recognised limitations: cost, invasive test with associated complication risk, sampling error and inter-interpreter variation (see Chapter 9). As a result there has been a growing interest in the development of alternative non-invasive markers that can be used in the diagnosis and monitoring of fibrosis in chronic liver disease. The majority of these tests have been developed in the last decade and are subject to on-going validation studies. In the future they are likely to be incorporated into routine diagnostic algorithms and clinical guidelines for the management of a number of common chronic liver diseases including NAFLD and chronic viral hepatitis (Tables 10.1 and 10.2). Their role is likely to be particularly valuable in primary care patients where they have the potential to accurately identify those individuals with advanced fibrosis who require specialist care in secondary or tertiary centres. It is estimated that ultimately non-invasive markers could reduce the need for liver biopsy by up to 80%.

Imaging

Transient ultrasound elastography (Fibroscan): Transient ultrasound elastography measures fibrosis by placing an ultrasound probe over the liver. A pulse generator contained within the probe produces a shear wave which spreads through the liver tissue and is detected by pulse-wave ultrasound imaging. The velocity of the shear wave is measured and correlates with the level of fibrosis. A measurement of greater than 7 kPa is indicative of significant fibrosis (Metavir grade F2-F4) and greater than 11-14 kPa is generally thought to be consistent with cirrhosis. Compared with a standard biopsy, Fibroscan can assess a much larger proportion of the liver parenchyma and therefore is associated with fewer sampling errors. Serial measurements are more acceptable to patients, making it an ideal test for monitoring treatment response (e.g. in chronic viral hepatitis; see Chapters 29 and 30). Although reproducibility is generally very good, it is reduced at the lower stages of fibrosis and in the presence of steatosis, significant ascites and /or inflammation.

Acoustic radiation force impulse: Acoustic radiation force impulse (ARFI) imaging is a further US-based tool that measures liver stiffness. It uses short-duration high-intensity acoustic pulses to induce a shear wave. Like in transient US elastography, the velocity of the wave correlates closely with amount of fibrosis. Limitations of the test are similar to those of Fibroscan.

Magnetic resonance imaging (see Chapter 8): High-quality cross-sectional imaging has an emerging role in the assessment of fibrosis. In cirrhosis, standard cross-sectional imaging by CT or MRI typically demonstrates parenchymal nodularity, an irregular liver border and signs of portal hypertension. However, earlier signs of fibrosis are often much more difficult to detect. Novel MR techniques such as diffusion-weighted MR, which measures the apparent diffusion coefficient of water, can detect early fibrogenesis. Magnetic resonance elastography (MRE), which combines elastography with MRI, has been shown to have a sensitivity of 92% and a specificity of 96% for detecting ≥F2 fibrosis. Compared with US elastography, MRE has the advantage of assessing the entire liver for fibrosis as well as providing simultaneous cross-sectional imaging; however, it is a longer test and considerably more expensive.

Serum markers

Products of fibrogenesis can be measured in the serum and used to detect the presence of liver fibrosis. Serum markers are broadly divided into direct and indirect markers. To improve the accuracy of these markers, they are increasingly being combined with other markers of liver function to improve their overall accuracy. Some panels use only direct markers (e.g. ELF), while others use only simple indirect markers (e.g. APRI) or a combination of both (e.g. Fibrotest, Hepascore).

Direct markers: Direct biomarkers of fibrosis include products of extracellular matrix synthesis or degradation, or cytokines and chemokines associated with fibrogenesis (e.g. procollagen types I and III), hyaluronic acid and tissue inhibitors of metalloproteinase. Algorithms combining direct markers include Fibrospect II, Shasta index and the ELF panel (Tables 10.1 and 10.2).

Indirect markers: Indirect markers detect alterations in hepatic function rather than fibrogenesis (e.g. serum aminotransferase levels, platelet count, INR, GGT, bilirubin, α2-macroglobulin, and α2-globulin (haptoglobin)). Many of these tests are performed routinely and are therefore easier to incorporate into clinical practice. Some of these algorithms (e.g. AST : ALT ratio; >1 is predictive of significant fibrosis), are relatively simple to calculate. Increasingly, the more complex algorithms are available through online calculators. The most studied indirect algorithms include APRI, Fibrotest/Fibrosure and Hepascore (Tables 10.1 and 10.2).

Limitations of serum markers: Some of the markers included in these algorithms reflect matrix turnover rather than collagen deposition and therefore can be falsely elevated by extrahepatic inflammatory activity. Alternatively, significant fibrogenesis may go undetected if there is minimal inflammation. Although these markers are increasingly reliable at detecting fibrosis they are recognised to correlate poorly with the level of fibrosis.

Breath tests

Breath tests have been used as non-invasive diagnostic tools in paediatric liver disease to detect conditions such as biliary atresia in infants. However, recently they have been explored as potential markers of fibrosis. Early clinical studies have shown 13C-methacetin has a sensitivity of 95% and a specificity of 74% for detecting fibrosis in NAFLD, although further validation studies are needed.

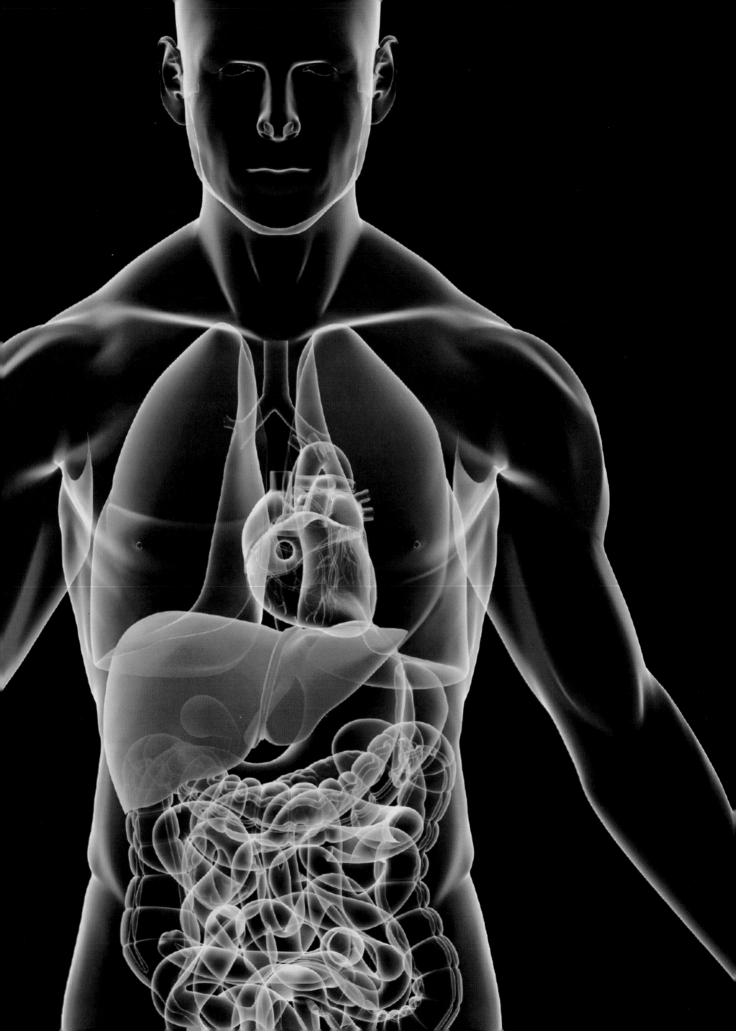

Clinical scenarios

Chapters

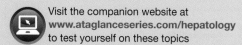

Visit the companion website at
www.ataglanceseries.com/hepatology
to test yourself on these topics

11 Asymptomatic abnormal LFTs

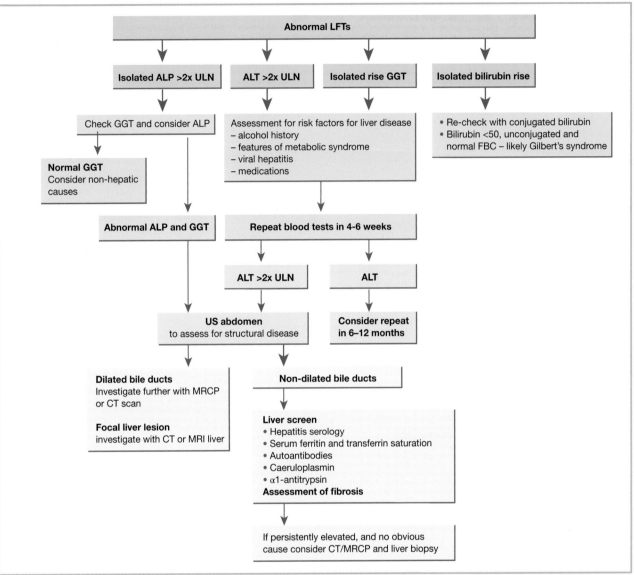

Patients often have abnormal liver function tests in the absence of hepatobiliary symptoms. Prevalence ranges from 6% to 21% of the UK population. We suggest an ALT >2 times the upper limit of normal (ULN) warrants further investigation as do patients with milder abnormalities but with significant risk factors for liver disease. This is a common clinical scenario in primary care.

Common causes of abnormal LFTs

1 Steatosis – alcohol or weight related;
2 Steatohepatitis – alcohol or weight related;
3 Viral hepatitis;
4 Iron overload/haemochromatosis;
5 Autoimmune liver disease;
6 Drug-induced liver disease;
7 Metabolic disease: Wilson's disease, α1-antitrypsin disease;
8 Chronic biliary disease: PSC, PBC;
9 Multisystemic disease.

Management

Involves the assessment of a underlying cause of abnormal LFTs and assessment of severity of liver damage. A lower threshold for investigations of abnormal asymptomatic LFTs is required in patients with familial risk factors, disease-related risk factors and those who are immunocompromised.

Comprehensive history and examination with specific attention to alcohol history and drug history (past and present). Risk factors for the metabolic syndrome: body mass index (BMI), hip : waist ratio, presence of diabetes, presence of hypertension, and fasting triglycerides.

A suggested algorithm for the investigation of asymptomatic LFTs is shown in the figure. Investigations and assessment should be made on an individual basis and be guided by the overall clinical context. Patients with persistent abnormal LFTs, abnormal imaging or a positive liver screen should be referred to secondary care.

Non-invasive liver screen

Blood tests

- Viral hepatitis: hepatitis B surface antigen (HBsAg), hepatitis C antibody;
- Iron induced liver disease: serum ferritin and transferrin saturations;
- Autoimmune liver disease: anti-smooth muscle antibody, anti-nuclear antibody, anti-mitochrondrial antibody and immunoglobulins;
- Wilson's disease: caeruloplasmin;
- α1-Antitrypsin genotype;
- Coeliac disease (e.g. tissue transglutaminase antibody).

Imaging

- *US liver and abdomen*: good screening tool for structural liver disease/biliary obstruction. If US findings are equivocal then further imaging of the external biliary tree maybe required (e.g. common bile duct stones). Further imaging maybe required and will be dictated by the non-invasive liver screen and US findings.
- *Fibroscan*: increasingly more available for rapid non-invasive assessment of fibrosis.

Assessment of severity

Routine LFTs are not particularly sensitive for early damage. An isolated increase in GGT rarely indicates significant liver disease.

- US scan for obvious signs of portal hypertension and cirrhosis;
- AST : ALT ratio >1;
- NAFLD fibrosis score (see Chapter 26);
- Score for viral hepatitis (APRI score);
- Fibrosis markers (if available) – see Chapter 10;
- Measurement of liver stiffness (Fibroscan or ARFI).

Integrated assessment pathways in primary and secondary care are being established and should be in accordance with national and local guidance.

Prognosis

The prognosis depends on underlying cause. In many individuals no definite cause can be found and it is often assumed abnormal LFTs are related to steatosis even with normal liver US scan. In the absence of risk factors for significant liver disease and a negative liver screen these individuals have a good prognosis.

12 Jaundice

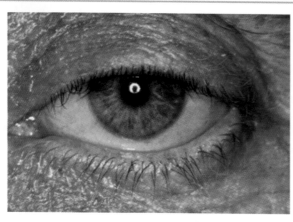

Figure 12-1 Jaundiced sclera.

Hepatology at a Glance, First Edition. Deepak Joshi, Geri Keane and Alison Brind.
© 2015 John Wiley & Sons, Ltd. Published 2015 by John Wiley & Sons, Ltd. Companion website: www.ataglanceseries.com/hepatology

Box 12.1 Unconjugated (indirect) hyperbilirubinaemia

Increased bilirubin production
- Intravascular/extravascular haemolysis
- Dyserythropoiesis

Impaired hepatic bilirubin uptake
- Heart failure
- Porto-systemic shunts
- Drugs

Impaired bilirubin conjugation
- Crigler-Najjar (Type I and II)
- Gilbert's syndrome
- Hyperthyroidism

Box 12.2 Conjugated (direct) hyperbilirubinaemia

Hepatocellular
- Any cause of liver injury/ disease

Cholestasis
- Intrahepatic cholestasis
  - Alcoholic hepatitis
  - Viral hepatitis
  - PBC
  - PSC
  - NASH
  - ICP
  - Dubin Johnson
  - Rotor syndrome
  - PFIC/BRIC/Alagille syndrome

- Extrahepatic cholestasis
  - Gallstones
  - Biliary strictures
  - Pancreatic malignancy
  - Cholangiocarcinoma
  - PSC
  - Lymph node compression
  - HIV-related cholangiopathy
  - Parasitic infections

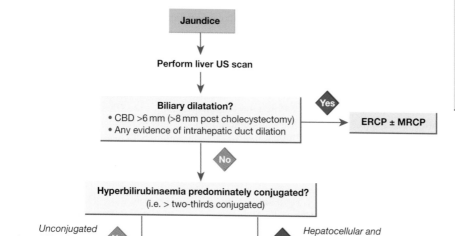

Figure 12-2 Investigation of jaundice.

Jaundice or hyperbilirubinaemia is the yellowing of the sclera and the skin (Figure 12.1) and occurs following deposition of bilirubin subcutaneously. It is usually clinically apparent >2 times ULN but can be more difficult to assess in darker skinned individuals.

Classification

Different classifications of jaundice exist (pre-hepatic, hepatic and post-hepatic). We recommend it should be divided primarily into unconjugated and conjugated hyperbilirubinaemia. See Chapter 7 for bilirubin production.

Unconjugated (indirect) hyperbilirubinaemia
Increased bilirubin production
• Intravascular or extravascular haemolysis (e.g. sickle cell anaemia, glucose-6-phosphate dehydrogenase deficiency, haemolytic uraemic syndrome, paroxysmal nocturnal haemoglobinuria, autoimmune-mediated haemolysis);
• Dyserythropoiesis.

Impaired hepatic bilirubin uptake
• Heart failure;
• Porto-systemic shunts;
• Drugs (e.g. rifampicin, probenecid).

Impaired hepatic bilirubin conjugation
• *Crigler–Najjar syndrome.* Type I: jaundice usually occurs immediately post birth and persists. Occurs due to no uridine diphosphoglucuronate-glucuronosyltransferase (UGT) activity. Patients are more likely to develop kernicterus (bilirubin encephalopathy). Treatment is with phototherapy and plasmapheresis. There is no response to phenobarbital. Liver transplantation is a curative option. Type II: also known as Arias syndrome. Associated with lower levels of hyperbilirubinaemia than type I. UGT is present but at reduced levels. Neurological complications are less common. Treatment is usually unnecessary but in those with symptoms related to jaundice, phenobarbital (induces residual UGT activity) can be used.
• *Gilbert's syndrome.* Affects 5% of the general population. More common in men. Occurs due to reduced *UGT1A1* activity. Inheritance is autosomal recessive. The genetic defect is within the promoter region of *UGT1A1* and occurs in patients who are homozygous for the defect. Episodes of jaundice tend to occur classically during illness or starvation. Patients are usually asymptomatic. The diagnosis can be made in patients with an unconjugated hyperbilirubinaemia in the absence of haemolysis and abnormal LFTs.
• *Hyperthyroidism.*

Conjugated (direct) hyperbilirubinaemia
Hepatocellular
Any cause of hepatoceullar injury or disease.

Cholestasis
Cholestasis refers to decreased bile flow and can be caused by defects in the transportation of bilirubin into the biliary system or by the physical obstruction of bile flow. Imaging of the biliary tree can help differentiate between extrahepatic and intrahepatic cholestasis.

Intrahepatic cholestasis: Any cause of hepatocellular injury or disease. Other causes include intestinal failure-associated liver disease (IFALD), intrahepatic cholestasis of pregnancy, progressive familial intrahepatic cholestasis (PFIC), benign recurrent intrahepatic cholestasis (BRIC), Dubin–Johnson syndrome, Rotor syndrome and Alagille syndrome.

Extrahepatic cholestasis (obstructive jaundice): The most common cause of a conjugated hyperbilirubinaemia. Causes include gallstones (most common cause), biliary strictures due to pancreatic malignancy, cholangiocarcinoma, acute and chronic pancreatitis, lymph node compression, PSC, HIV-related cholangiopathy (rare), parasitic infections (e.g. *Ascaris lumbricoides*, liver flukes).

Rare causes of intrahepatic cholestasis
Dubin-Johnson syndrome
A benign condition which occurs due to a defect in the ability of hepatocytes to secrete bilirubin (mutation in the canalicular multidrug resistance protein 2, MRP2). Liver classically appears 'black' on biopsy. No treatment is required.

Rotor syndrome
Also a benign condition which occurs due to a defect in the reuptake of conjugated bilirubin by hepatocytes. LFTs are normal and liver histology is also normal. No specific treatment is required.

Progressive familial intrahepatic cholestasis
Group of disorders characterised by a defect in the secretion of bile. PFIC type 1 (Byler's disease) first described in the Amish population.
Characteristically, GGT is normal. Gene defect is related to the FIC1 locus on chromosome 18q21-q22 encoding an ATPase (ATP8B1). PFIC type 2 occurs due to mutation in bile salt export pump (BSEP) on chromosome 2. PFIC type 3 occurs due to mutation in MDR3 gene on chromosome. GGT is usually elevated. Usually present in infancy or childhood. Associated with intractable itch and progressive liver failure.

Benign recurrent intrahepatic cholestasis
A few variants exist. Autosomal inheritance. Occurs from infancy to late adulthood. Characterised by recurrent attacks. Raised ALP, normal transaminases and GGT. Associated with intrahepatic cholestasis of pregnancy and use of the oral contraceptive pill. Supportive treatment.

Alagille syndrome
Autosomal dominant. Occurs due to microdeletion of 20p12 gene corresponding to JAG1. Characterised by a paucity of interlobular bile ducts. Associated with cardiac anomalies, butterfly vertebrae and dysmorphic facies (triangular face, high forehead, saddle-shaped nasal bridge).

13 Portal hypertension

Pre-hepatic PHT

Oesophageal varices

Portal vein thrombosis

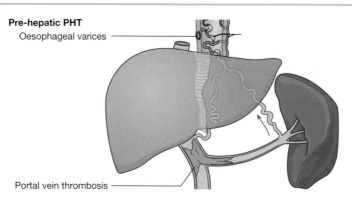

Intrahepatic PHT

Spleen often markedly enlarged

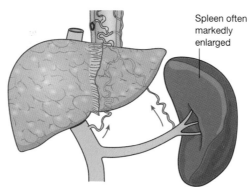

Post-hepatic PHT

Tricuspid incompetence

Thrombosis of hepatic veins (Budd–Chiari syndrome)

Hepatomegaly

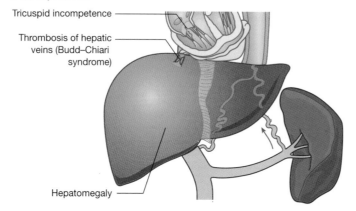

Table 13-1 Interpretation of portal venous pressure studies.

		WHVP	FHVP	HVPG
Prehepatic (e.g. portal vein thrombus)		Normal	Normal	Normal
Intrahepatic	**Presinusoidal** (e.g. schistosomaisis)	Normal	Normal	Normal
	Sinusoidal (e.g. cirrhosis)	Increased	Increased	Increased
Posthepatic	**Budd-Chiari syndrome** – hepatic vein cannot be cannulated due to clot	N/A	N/A	N/A
	Other posthepatic causes (e.g. right heart failure, IVC webs)	Increased	Increased	Normal

Hepatology at a Glance, First Edition. Deepak Joshi, Geri Keane and Alison Brind.
© 2015 John Wiley & Sons, Ltd. Published 2015 by John Wiley & Sons, Ltd. Companion website: www.ataglanceseries.com/hepatology

Portal hypertension (PHT) is defined as a hepatic venous pressure gradient (HVPG) of >5 mmHg. Complications rarely occur as long as the HVPG is <12 mmHg.

Pathophysiology

The initial factor in the development of PHT is venous compression and/or obstruction leading to an increase in vascular resistance. This can occur at the pre-hepatic, sinusoidal or post-hepatic levels. In cirrhosis, it occurs at the level of the sinusoid and affects the hepatic microcirculation. In a cirrhotic liver, on-going fibrogenesis results in the release of a number of endogenous factors such as endothelin-1, α-adrenergic stimulus and angiotensin II. These factors cause vasoconstriction and increased vascular resistance. In addition, production of nitric oxide, a vasodilator, is reduced. Another major component in the aetiology of increased PHT is the increased portal venous inflow, which occurs as a result of concomitant splanchnic arteriolar vasodilatation.

Location and causes of resistance

Pre-hepatic causes
- Portal or splenic vein thrombosis;
- Congenital atresia or stenosis of portal vein;
- Extrinsic compression of portal vein (e.g. pancreatic tumour);
- Splanchnic arteriovenous fistula.

Intrahepatic causes
Predominantly pre-sinusoidal:
- Schistosomiasis;
- Non-cirrhotic portal fibrosis (NCPF)/idiopathic PHT;
- Primary biliary cirrhosis;
- Nodular regenerative hyperplasia – due to compression of the intrahepatic portal venules; and
- Hepatic metastasis, myeloproliferative diseases or granulomatous diseases (e.g. sarcoidosis or TB) due to infiltration or compression of the intrahepatic portal venules.

   Predominantly sinusoidal:
- Cirrhosis; and
- Acute alcoholic hepatitis.

Post-hepatic causes
- Budd–Chiari syndrome or IVC thrombosis;
- Right-sided heart failure, constrictive pericarditis or severe tricuspid regurgitation;
- IVC webs.

Consequences of sustained portal hypertension

Portosystemic collaterals:
The portal vein carries approximately 1500 mL/min of blood from the small and large bowel, spleen and the stomach to the liver. If there is sustained PHT, veins dilate and collaterals develop at communications between the portal and systemic circulations (e.g. oesophagogastric, rectal, duodenal, stomal and retroperitoneal). Oesophagogastric varices are of particular importance because of their risk of rupture, precipitating a gastrointestinal hemorrhage (see Chapter 14).

Clinical signs and symptoms of PHT
- Varices;
- Ascites (less likely in pre-sinusoidal PHT);
- Hepatorenal syndrome or spontaneous bacterial peritonitis;
- Splenomegaly;
- Caput medusa;
- Portal cavernoma on imaging;
- Jaundice (portal hypertensive bilopathy);
- Hepatic encephalopathy (due to portosystemic shunts).

Diagnosis

The gold standard method of diagnosing PHT is by measuring the HVPG. HVPG is a measure of portal (sinusoidal) pressure. It is measured by performing portal venous pressure studies (see Table 13.1). This requires catheterisation of a hepatic vein via the jugular or femoral vein. A wedged hepatic vein pressure (WHVP) is then obtained, from which the free hepatic vein pressure (FHVP) is subtracted to calculate HVPG (normally 3–5 mmHg). Portal venous pressure studies can also be used to determine of the site of obstruction in PHT (see Table 13.1).

Management and prognosis

HVPG is an important predictor of a patient's overall prognosis in advanced liver disease. It also predicts the likelihood of developing varices and gastrointestinal haemorrhage. HVPG can be measured serially to monitor response to therapy and progression of liver disease. However, it is an invasive test and is rarely performed outside of specialist centres. If HVPG can be reduced to <12 mmHg by pharmacotherapy (e.g. non-selective beta-blockers or interventional radiological/surgical shunts, e.g. TIPS), more than 90% of cirrhotic patients will not develop variceal haemorrhage or ascites.

Non-cirrhotic portal hypertension: If signs and symptoms of PHT occur in the absence of liver cirrhosis, non-cirrhotic portal hypertension (NCPH) should be considered. Although NCPH is rare in Europe and North America, it is a common cause of PHT in Asia and sub-Saharan Africa.

   NCPH is a heterogeneous group of diseases that arise largely as a result of pre-sinusoidal obstruction. Common causes include NCPF, also known as idiopathic PHT, hepatoportal sclerosis, and obliterative venopathy, and extrahepatic portal vein obstruction (EHPVO). Rarer causes include schistosomiasis, congenital hepatic fibrosis and nodular regenerative hyperplasia. The prevalence of NCPF in HIV-positive patients is increasing due to the use of certain highly active antiretroviral therapy (HAART) medications (e.g. didanosine). NCPH commonly presents with variceal haemorrhage. Splenomegaly is a common finding on clinical examination. NCPH is managed similarly to cirrhotic portal hypertension with pharmacotherapy or surgical portosystemic shunting. Prognosis is better than for cirrhotic PHT.

14 Variceal bleeding

Sengstaken–Blakemore tube (SBT)

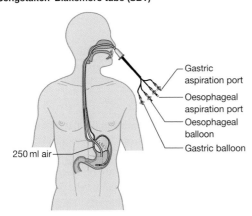

Gastric
aspiration port

Oesophageal
aspiration port

Oesophageal
balloon

Gastric balloon

250 ml air

Performed under sedation and ideally general anaesthesia. Insert SBT to the limit of tube and inflate gastric balloon with 250 mL air. Clamp the gastric balloon port and pull back until resistance is met and secure tube (approx. 28–30 cm at the incisors). If bleeding continues apply traction to the tube by attaching a 500-mL bag of fluid or consider inflating the oesophageal balloon. Aspirate gastric and oesophageal ports frequently. Position can be confirmed by X-ray. Aim to deflate and remove SBT within 18 hours.

Figure 14-1   Rescue therapy.

Oesophageal self-expanding metal stent (SEMS)

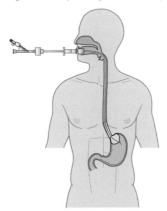

The SX-Ella Danis stent (Ella-CS, Hradec Kralove, Czech Republic) is a removable, covered SEMS that can be deployed in the lower oesophagus over an endoscopically placed guidewire. The stent controls bleeding by tamponade of varices and can be left in place for up to 2 weeks

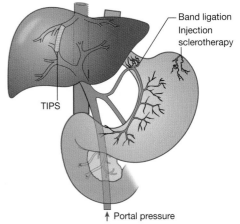

Band ligation
Injection
sclerotherapy

TIPS

↑ Portal pressure

Figure 14-2   Definitive endoscopic or radiological management.

Table 14-1   Contraindications to TIPS placement.

Absolute	Relative
Primary prevention of variceal bleeding	HCC
Congestive heart failure	Obstruction of all hepatic veins
Multiple hepatic cysts	Portal vein thrombosis
Systemic infection	Severe coagulopathy (INR >5)
Unrelieved biliary obstruction	Thrombocytopenia (<20x10^9/L)
Progressive renal failure	Moderate pulmonary hypertension
Severe pulmonary hypertension	Hepatic encephalopathy (HE > Grade 2)

Oesophageal varices (OV) are present in one-third of patients with compensated cirrhosis and two-thirds of those with decompensated cirrhosis at diagnosis. Of cirrhotic patients, 5–7% develop OV annually. Up to one-third of those with OV will also have gastric varices (GV). Once established, small OV progress to large OV at a rate of approximately 8% per year. Risk factors for variceal rupture include size of varix, severity of liver disease, sepsis, HCC and elevated HVPG. OV have a risk of bleeding of approximately 25% at 2 years. Varices account for 11% of all gastrointestinal bleeds in the UK but 70% of bleeds in cirrhotic patients. Acute variceal haemorrhage is associated with 15–20% mortality. Overall mortality in all patients with OV is estimated to be 20–64% at 1 year.

Diagnosis and surveillance

A screening gastroscopy for varices is recommended in all patients with cirrhosis at diagnosis and then every 2–3 years in compensated cirrhosis and annually in decompensation. Non-invasive markers have been investigated as alternatives to surveillance endoscopy, but none are currently sufficiently reliable. Patients

Hepatology at a Glance, First Edition. Deepak Joshi, Geri Keane and Alison Brind.
© 2015 John Wiley & Sons, Ltd. Published 2015 by John Wiley & Sons, Ltd. Companion website: www.ataglanceseries.com/hepatology

already taking non-selective beta-blockers (NSBB) do not require surveillance gastroscopy.

Endoscopic grading of OV

Table 14.2

British Society of Gastroenterology	American Association for the Study of Liver Diseases
Grade 1 (small): collapse with air insufflation	Small: minimally elevated veins
Grade 2 (medium): not collapsible	Medium: tortuous veins < one-third of the lumen
Grade 3 (large): occluding oesophageal lumen	Large: >one-third of the lumen

Management

Pre-primary prophylaxis

For patients with compensated cirrhosis, without varices, pre-primary prophylaxis with NSBB is not thought to prevent the subsequent development of varices.

Primary prophylaxis

Primary prophylaxis is defined as the prevention of variceal haemorrhage in those with OV that have not bled. Primary prophylaxis is recommended for all patients with large OV, and those with moderate OV with 'red sign' or Child–Pugh B or C cirrhosis. Prophylaxis can be by pharmacological therapy with NSBBs (e.g. propranolol or carvidolol) or by endoscopic band ligation (EBL). NSBB act by decreasing cardiac output and increasing splanchnic vasoconstriction, therefore reducing portal pressure. The dose of NSBB is titrated up until the heart rate decreases by 25% from baseline (side effects include postural hypotension). Once NSBB prophylaxis is initiated, lifelong treatment is advised. Although EBL may provide a greater reduction in the risk of variceal haemorrhage compared to NSBB, there is no additional survival advantage and potentially more frequent complications (e.g. post-EBL bleeding). Therefore, EBL as part of primary prophylaxis is only recommended in those who are intolerant of NSBB or have Child–Pugh C cirrhosis with large varices. Combination therapy with NSBB and EBL has no additional clinical benefit and potentially greater side effects.

Management of acute variceal haemorrhage and secondary prophylaxis

Medical management: Variceal haemorrhage is a medical emergency. Patients should be treated in a high dependency area (e.g. HDU or ITU). IV access should be established promptly and fluid resuscitation commenced with the aim of achieving haemodynamic stability. In torrential bleeding, insertion of a Sengstaken–Blakemore tube (SBT; see Figure 14.1) can obtain temporary control of the haemorrhage. Blood transfusions should be administered to maintain a haemoglobin level >7 g/dL. Excessive transfusions have been associated with increases in HVPG, rebleeding and increased mortality. Prophylactic antibiotics (e.g. 1–2 g ceftriaxone) reduce the risk of rebleeding, infection and decrease mortality. Terlipressin (a synthetic vasopressin analogue) or other somatostatin analogues reduce HVPG and should be commenced promptly and continued for 2–5 days post-variceal haemorrhage.

Endoscopic therapy: Without treatment variceal bleeding stops spontaneously in half of cases but rebleeding is common (30–40%). Gastroscopy with EBL is therefore recommended within 12 hours of admission and following appropriate resuscitation and anaesthetic support in unstable patients. Sclerotherapy is an option when EBL is not feasible. Further gastroscopy with or without EBL should be performed 2–4 weekly until OV have been obliterated.

Rescue therapy: In the 10–20% of cases when medical and endoscopic therapy fails to control bleeding or recurrent bleeding occurs. Management options include the following:

• Transjugular intrahepatic portosystemic shunt (TIPS): a metal stent is inserted between the hepatic and portal veins reducing HVPG (see Figure 14.1). Early use of TIPS for acute variceal haemorrhage in high-risk patients (Child–Pugh C cirrhosis or Child–Pugh B with persistent bleeding at endoscopy) has been shown to reduce overall mortality and rebleeding rates. Complications include HE in one-third. Post-TIPS HE responds to medical treatment in most cases.

• Balloon tamponade with an SBT (see Figure 14.1) can temporally control haemorrhage in patients while awaiting more definitive therapy (e.g. endoscopic therapy or TIPS).

• Endoscopic insertion of a self-expanding fully covered oesophageal stent (e.g. SX-Ella Danis stent is an alternative to SBT or early TIPS; see Figure 14.1).

• Surgical options (rarely required): surgical portosystemic shunting, oesophageal devascularisation or liver transplantation.

Gastric varices: 5–33% of patients with portal hypertension will have GV. GV are a rare cause of gastrointestinal haemorrhage in cirrhotic patients (5–10% cases). However, bleeding from GV is often severe and survival is worse than in haemorrhage due to OV. GV can be treated endoscopically with injection of N-butyl-2-cyanoacrylate, isobutyl-2-cyanoacrylate or thrombin. Meticulous adherence to technique is crucial to prevent damage to endoscopes by tissue adhesives. Complications include glue embolus to the portal vein, coronary artery, spleen, lungs or brain. TIPS can also be used as an alternative first line therapy or as second line therapy in the management of GV haemorrhage. In specialist centres, if a TIPS fails to control haemorrhage interventional radiologists may consider balloon-occluded retrograde transvenous obliteration (BRTO) where ethanolamine oleate is injected retrogradely into the GV.

Ectopic varices: Bleeding can occur from rectal, peristomal and duodenal varices. Management is with pharmacological therapy (e.g. terlipressin) in the acute situation, followed by NSBB long-term or TIPS if these measures fail.

⑮ Ascites

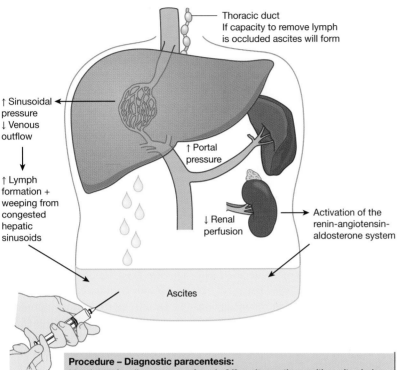

Thoracic duct
If capacity to remove lymph
is occluded ascites will form

↑ Sinusoidal
pressure
↓ Venous
outflow

↑ Lymph
formation +
weeping from
congested
hepatic
sinusoids

↑ Portal
pressure

↓ Renal
perfusion

Activation of the
renin-angiotensin-
aldosterone system

Ascites

**Box 15-1 Common causes
of ascites**

Portal hypertension
Cirrhosis (75%)
Alcoholic hepatitis
Acute liver failure
Hepatic veno-occlusive disease,
    e.g. Budd-Chiari syndrome
Congestive heart failure
Constrictive pericarditis

Hypoalbuminemia
Nephrotic syndrome
Protein-losing enteropathy
Severe malnutrition

Peritoneal disease
Malignant ascites (10%)
Ovarian disease (benign and
    malignant tumours)
Infectious or granulomatous
    peritonitis (e.g. TB, sarcoid)

Other
Hypothyroidism
Pancreatic ascites e.g. ruptured
    pseudocyst or disrupted duct
Nephrotic syndrome
Chylous ascites e.g. lymphoma
    or intestinal lymphangiectasia

Procedure – Diagnostic paracentesis:
Mandatory for all new cases of grade 2/3 ascites or those with ascites being
admitted to hospital. Proceed by ascertaining the upper level of ascites by
percussion in right lower quadrant. Clean skin and aspirate 20mls of ascites
via a needle and syringe. The fluid should be straw coloured, bloodstaining
suggests malignancy and cloudy fluid suggests infection. Send sample for
analysis as outlined opposite

Box 15-2

Transudate (SAAG >11g/l)	Exudate (SAAG <11g/l)
• Cirrhosis and portal hypertension – SAAG > 11g/l = 97% sensitivity for portal hypertension • Congestive cardiac failure • Hypothyroidism • Hepatic vein occlusion	• Peritoneal carcinomatosis • Infection (e.g. TB) • Pancreatic ascites • Nephrotic syndrome • Serositis • Chylous ascites • Low protein states e.g. kwashiorkor

Hepatology at a Glance, First Edition. Deepak Joshi, Geri Keane and Alison Brind.
© 2015 John Wiley & Sons, Ltd. Published 2015 by John Wiley & Sons, Ltd. Companion website: www.ataglanceseries.com/hepatology

Ascites

Ascites is the defined as an accumulation of fluid within the peritoneal cavity. Common causes are outlined in Box 15.1.

Investigations

Laboratory tests: full blood count (FBC), urea and electrolytes (U&E), LFT, C-reactive protein (CRP), clotting and urinary sodium. Consider also amylase, brain natriuretic peptide (BNP), TB assessment or rheumatoid factor depending on suspected underlying aetiology.

Abdominal ultrasound: Evaluates liver parenchyma for nodularity consistent with cirrhosis, presence of HCC and vessel patency. In large volume ascites the abdominal wall can be marked for drainage.

Diagnostic paracentesis (see figure) + ascitic fluid analysis:

• *Albumin:* the serum ascites albumin gradient (SAAG) is useful in determining aetiology (see Box 15.2).

• SAAG = erum albuminascitic fluid albumin.

• *Protein:* <15 g/L + Child–Pugh C cirrhosis is associated with an increased risk of SBP – consider long-term antibiotic prophylaxis (e.g. 400 mg/day norfloxacin).

• *WCC:* >250 neutrophils/mm^3 is indicative of spontaneous bacterial peritonitis (SBP).

• *Culture and sensitivities* ± AFB (if TB likely). NB: inoculate blood culture bottles at the bedside.

• *Cytology:* especially when malignancy is suspected.

• *Amylase:* if pancreatic aetiology likely.

• *Glucose and LDH:* decreased glucose and increased LDH is suggestive of secondary bacterial peritontis.

Extrahepatic investigations: If liver function tests are normal consider cross-sectional imaging to exclude malignancy, ECG and echocardiogram to exclude congestive cardiac failure or constrictive pericarditis and/or a 24-hour urinary protein collection or protein: creatinine ratio to assess for nephrotic syndrome.

Definitions of ascites in liver disease

Uncomplicated ascites: Ascites that is not infected or associated with the development of hepato-renal syndrome (HRS).

Refractory ascites:

• *Diuretic-resistant ascites:* unresponsive to diuretic treatment;

• *Diuretic-intractable ascites:* therapeutic complications precluding further treatment.

Pathogenesis

There are two key factors involved in the pathogenesis of ascites in liver disease: portal hypertension (see Chapter 13) and sodium and water retention. Sodium retention is thought to occur due to arterial vasodilatation causing renal hypoperfusion, which triggers the activation of the renin–angiotensin system and aldosterone release. Aldosterone hypersecretion is one of the mechanisms by which sodium and water reabsorption occurs at the distal tubule in cirrhosis.

Grading and management of uncomplicated ascites

Table 15.1

Grade	Definition	Treatment
1	Minimal ascites only detectable by ultrasound	No treatment
2	Moderate ascites with distension of the abdomen	Restriction of sodium intake (<1.5 g/day) and fluid (<1.5 L/day) and diuretics
3	Gross ascites with marked abdominal distension	Large volume paracentesis followed by sodium restriction and diuretics (unless refractory)

Diet: Moderate restriction of salt intake is recommended (80–120 mmol/day or 4.6–6.9 g salt/day). Fluid restriction is widely practised but of limited efficacy.

Diuretics: In new onset grade 2 ascites, commence 100 mg/day spironolactone (aldosterone antagonist). Consider a lower dose in those with deranged renal function. Check potassium before commencing diuretic therapy. Increase spironolactone by 100 mg every 7 days to a maximum of 400 mg/day. Aim for 0.5 kg/day (without oedema) and 1 kg/day (with oedema) weight loss. If patients do not respond to diuretic therapy (<2 kg/week weight loss) or develop hyperkalaemia, furosemide can be added staring at 40 mg/day increasing in increments to a maximum of 160 mg/day. If patients remain unresponsive, measure urinary sodium and if less than 30 mmol/L discontinue diuretics and consider alternative management (see Chapter 16).

Complications of diuretic therapy: During the initiation and titration of diuretics patients should be monitored closely and U&Es checked every few days. If sodium falls to <120 mmol/L or patients develop HE or they notice muscle cramps or have a significant deterioration in renal function, stop all diuretic therapy immediately. If hypokalaemia (potassium <3 mmol/L) occurs stop furosemide and if hyperkalaemia (potassium >6 mmol/L) develops stop spironolactone. After the initial episode of ascites has been successfully treated, diuretics should be titrated to the minimum dose required to prevent recurrence of ascites.

Therapeutic paracentesis: In patients with grade 3 ascites large volume paracentesis (LVP) is advocated as part of initial management. LVP should be completed in one session, with the drain removed after 6 hours. Concomitant albumin replacement (8 g/L drained) is advised to prevent circulatory dysfunction. Post LVP, diuretic therapy should be commenced and titrated to prevent recurrence.

Drugs: Where possible avoid NSAIDs, aminoglycoside antibiotics (e.g. gentamicin) and drugs that decrease renal blood flow (e.g. ACE inhibitors) and angiotensin II antagonists which may precipitate HRS.

Liver transplantation: The presence of ascites is associated with a mortality of 50% at 2 years and once refractory increases to 50% at 6 months. Early transplant assessment is therefore recommended.

Management of complications of ascites

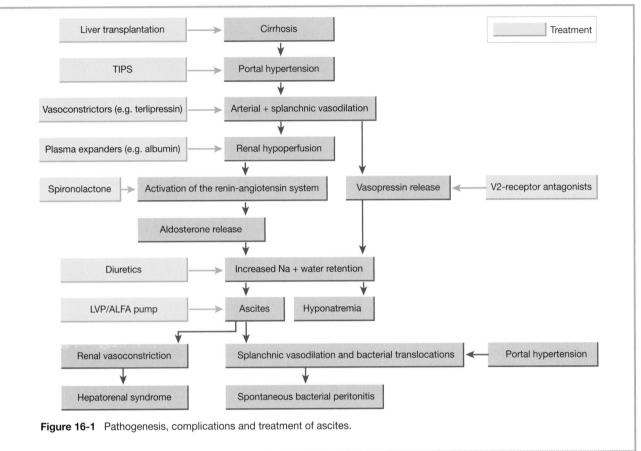

Figure 16-1 Pathogenesis, complications and treatment of ascites.

Hepatology at a Glance, First Edition. Deepak Joshi, Geri Keane and Alison Brind.
© 2015 John Wiley & Sons, Ltd. Published 2015 by John Wiley & Sons, Ltd. Companion website: www.ataglanceseries.com/hepatology

Management of refractory ascites

Recurrent large volume paracentesis (LVP): LVP is the primary therapy for patients with refractory ascites. It is often performed as a day case procedure, with albumin replacement (8 g/L of ascites removed) as and when patients become symptomatic.

Transjugular intrahepatic portosystemic shunt: Prevents ascites formation by reducing the HVPG (see Chapter 14 for procedure description). Compared with LVP, ascites reoccurs less frequently following TIPS but there is no additional survival advantage. Following TIPS, ascites improves in 38–84% of patients, but resolution may be slow and diuretics or LVP may be required in the initial stages. Common indications for TIPS include frequent LVP, loculated ascites and recurrent hydrothrorax. Surgical portovenous shunts are an alternative to TIPS but rarely used as associated with greater morbidity.

Liver transplantation: Refractory ascites with or without complications is associated with a very poor prognosis and is an indication to consider liver transplant assessment.

Novel therapies: The ALFApump® system (Sequana Medical AG) is a surgically implantable device that continuously pumps ascites from the abdomen into the bladder, where it is eliminated through normal urination. Its efficacy is currently being evaluated through ongoing clinical trials.

Complication of ascites
Spontaneous bacterial peritonitis

Aetiology: Portal hypertension causes splanchnic vasodilatation, bowel wall oedema and increased permeability leading to bacteria translocation from the intestine to the ascites. Gram-negative bacteria (e.g. *Escherichia coli*) translocate more efficiently than Gram-positive bacteria or anaerobes.

Presentation: Typical symptoms of sepsis are often absent. Diagnostic paracentesis is recommended in all patients being admitted to hospital with ascites or who develop signs of decompensation to exclude SBP.

Definitions:
- *SBP:* >250/mm³ neutrophils in ascitic fluid. Fluid culture is often negative and not essential for diagnosis.
- *Bacterascites:* Ascitic neutrophil count of <250/mm³ but positive ascitic fluid cultures. If there are signs of sepsis, commence treatment immediately; otherwise, repeat a diagnostic paracentesis.
- *Spontaneous bacterial pleural empyema* – infected hydrothorax: pleural fluid neutrophil count >250/mm³ + positive culture. Pleural neutrophil count >500/mm³ with negative culture. Treatment as per SBP.
- *Secondary bacterial peritonitis* is defined by a surgically treatable source of infection (e.g. perforated viscous or perinephric abscess). It is suggested by a low glucose, raised LDH and persistently elevated neutrophil count in the ascitic fluid despite treatment. If suspected a CT and surgical opinion are advised.

Management: Broad-spectrum antibiotics (e.g. third-generation cephalosporin such as cefotaxime) and albumin (1.5 g/kg at diagnosis and 1 g/kg on day 3). The administration of albumin decreases the likelihood of HRS and improves survival. Antibiotics are generally continued for 5–10 days. Serial diagnostic paracenteses are used to monitor resolution (ascitic neutrophil count <250 mm³ and culture negative). No response to treatment (10% patients) is usually because of resistant organisms or secondary bacterial peritonitis. In these cases management should be amended accordingly.

Prophylaxis: Following an episode of spontaneous bacterial peritonitis prophylactic antibiotics (e.g. 400 mg/day norfloxacin) are advised to prevent recurrence.

Hepato-renal syndrome

Major diagnostic criteria: Acute or chronic liver disease, decreased GFR (creatinine >133 μmol/L), absence of other causes of renal failure (e.g. sepsis, drugs or renal parenchymal disease), no sustained improvement in glomerular filtration rate (GFR) with fluid challenge, normal renal US, proteinuria <0.5 g/day (Chapter 17).

Classification: The International Ascites Club revised their definition of HRS in 2007 and divide it clinically into two types. Type 1 HRS occurs acutely and is characterised by a rapid decline in renal function, often in association with an episode of decompensation secondary to SBP. Type 2 HRS is characterised by a more chronic, indolent reduction in renal function, which is associated with refractory ascites.

Management:
- Diligent fluid balance management. Stop all diuretics.
- Terlipressin (0.5–1 mg/4–6-hourly) + albumin. Complete response = creatinine <133 μmol/L. If creatinine does not decrease by one-quarter at day 3 terlipressin should be titrated up to a maximum of 2 mg/4-hourly. If a complete response is not seen at 14 days discontinue treatment. Terlipressin therapy should be used with care in patients with ischaemic heart disease. While on treatment, monitor daily for signs of digital or splanchnic ischaemia and adjust dose accordingly. If HRS occurs on stopping therapy, treatment can be recommenced as above.
- Renal replacement therapy: may be required in those who do not respond to medical management and who fulfil criteria for renal support.
- Liver transplantation: as in all forms of refractory ascites, transplant assessment is advised. In those requiring dialysis for >3 months prior to transplantation, combined liver and renal transplants are often required.

Hyponatraemia

Aetiology: In cirrhosis, reduced arterial blood volume causes vasopressin hypersecretion and disproportionate water retention, a dilutional hyponatraemia and hypervolaemia (see figure).

Management:
- Fluid restriction to <1 L/day is only effective in a limited number of patients but may prevent progression of hyponatraemia. Should be used with caution due to risk of hypovolaemia. No role for hypertonic saline replacement but albumin may have some effect.
- V2 receptor antagonists (vaptans, e.g. tolvaptan) act on the distal tubule of the kidney to increase solute-free water excretion. This new therapy is currently licenced for use in severe hyponatraemia (sodium <125 mmol/L) in some countries.
- Serum sodium should be corrected slowly (<8–10 mmol/day) to prevent osmotic demyelination syndrome.

Hyponatraemia may also occur as a result of over-diuresis causing hyponatraemia with hypovolaemia. These patients are best managed by stopping diuretics and commencing slow IV crystalloid.

17 Renal dysfunction in cirrhosis

Box 17-1 Causes of renal dysfunction in cirrhosis

- Acute kidney injury
- Hepatorenal syndrome
- Structural renal diseases complicating primary liver disease
- Renal dysfunction and liver disease occurring together as part of a systemic illness
- Chronic kidney disease co-existing in a patient with cirrhosis

Box 17-2 Renal screen

- FBC, blood film, coagulation screen
- U&Es, bone profile (calcium and profile), glucose
- Septic screen
- Myoglobin and CK – if rhabdomyolysis is being considered
- Renal tract ultrasound – size and shape of kidneys, patency or renal arteries, evidence of hydronephrosis?
- Urine
  - Dipstick
  - Osmolality
  - Microscopy – for casts
  - Culture
  - Protein – 24 hour collection or spot protein/creatinine ratio
  - Bence Jones – if myeloma is considered
- Complement (C3, C4)
- Anti-GBM – Goodpasture's disease
- ENA, ANA, ANCA, – ANA positive in SLE and other connective tissue diseases
- Rheumatoid factor, immunoglobulins, protein electrophoresis
- Other
  - Leptospirosis
  - ASOT
  - Syphilis
  - HIV, CMV, VZV, hepatitis serology

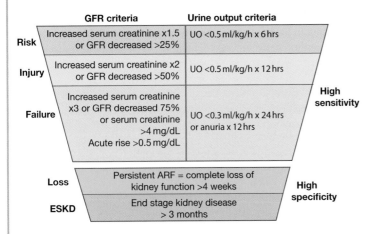

Figure 17-1 RIFLE (R, renal risk; I, injury; F, failure; L, loss; E, end-stage renal disease) diagnostic criteria.
Source: *Bellomo R et al., Crit Care (2004).*

Box 17-3 International ascites club diagnostic criteria for hepatorenal syndrome

- Cirrhosis with ascites
- Serum creatinine >133 μmol/L (1.5 mg/dL)
- No improvement in serum creatinine (decrease to a level of ≤133 μmol/L or 1.5 mg/dL) after at least 2 days of diuretic withdrawal and volume expansion with albumin.
  The recommended dose of albumin is 1 g/kg body weight/day up to a maximum of 100 g/day
- Absence of shock
- Absence of parenchymal kidney disease as indicated by proteinuria >500 mg/day, microhaematuria (>50 red blood cells/high power field) and/or abnormal renal ultrasonography

Renal dysfunction in cirrhosis

The development of renal dysfunction in patients with cirrhosis is associated with increased morbidity and mortality. Renal dysfunction in the setting of cirrhosis can be classified as: (i) acute kidney injury (AKI); (ii) hepato-renal syndrome (HRS); (iii) structural renal diseases complicating primary liver disease (e.g. IgA nephropathy, cryoglobulinaemia); (iv) renal dysfunction and liver disease occurring together as part of systemic illnesses (e.g. polycystic liver and kidney disease); and (v) chronic kidney disease (CKD) coexisting in a patient with cirrhosis. Type 1 HRS is regarded as a specific form of AKI.

Assessment of renal function

Serum creatinine is a poor marker of GFR and insensitive to a decline in GFR in cirrhotic patients. Serum creatinine levels are reduced by nearly 50% due to decreased hepatic production from creatine, malnutrition, loss of muscle mass and an increase in the volume of extracellular fluid (e.g. ascites). In the context of hyperbilirubinaemia, serum creatinine levels may underestimate the degree of renal impairment. In addition, serum urea levels may also be reduced due to decreased muscle mass. Serum biomarkers such as cystatin C and neutrophil gelatinase-associated lipocalin remain experimental.

Acute kidney injury

AKI affects 20% of patients with cirrhosis and ascites who are admitted to hospital. It often occurs in conjunction with other complications of cirrhosis (e.g. variceal bleeding). The RIFLE criteria (R, renal risk; I, injury; F, failure; L, loss of kidney function; E, end-stage renal disease) has been well validated in non-cirrhotic cohorts and stratifies acute renal dysfunction into grades of severity using changes in serum creatinine and/or urine output. The AKIN (Acute Kidney Injury Network) criteria is also well validated. AKI is associated with increased mortality and mortality rates increase as AKI parameters worsen.

Chronic kidney disease

CKD occurs in approximately 1% of all cirrhotic patients. Cirrhotic patients have poorer outcomes than patients with similar aetiologies and severity of renal dysfunction. CKD is defined as a GFR <60 mL/min for more than 3 months using the Modification of Diet in Renal Disease (MDRD6) formula. Type 2 HRS should therefore be regarded as a form of CKD. Patients with cirrhosis and CKD thought to be unrelated to the underlying liver aetiology may need assessment for joint liver–kidney transplantation.

Management of renal dysfunction in cirrhosis

All cirrhotic patients with renal dysfunction should have a comprehensive renal screen performed at their index presentation. (see Box 17.2). A renal tract ultrasound is required to assess the size and shape of the kidneys and exclude an obstructive cause. Nephrology input may be required.

1 *Assessment of fluid status.* Correct hypovolaemia. Avoid 5% dextrose in patients with ascites. Human albumin solution 4.5% or 20% can be used as volume expanders. Patients may require urinary catheterisation. Strict input–output documentation.

2 *Urinary analysis.* Bed-side urine dipstick may identify proteinuria or haematuria and therefore an intrinsic cause of renal dysfunction (e.g. nephrotic/nephritic syndrome).

3 *Correct electrolytes.* Hyponatraemia is common especially in patients with ascites. Judicious use of saline in the context of hyponatraemia may be needed. Correct hypo-/hyperkalaemia, Hypo-/hypercalcaemia, hypo-/hyperphosphataemia.

4 *Septic screen.* Renal dysfunction may be precipitated or exacerbated by sepsis. Patients require blood cultures, urinary microscopy culture and sensitivity, chest X-ray and a diagnostic ascitic tap (if ascites is present). Renal dosing of antibiotics may be required given the degree of renal impairment.

5 *Stop all nephrotoxic drugs.* Careful review of the patient's medications is required. Diuretics may need to stopped temporarily.

6 *Consider abdominal paracentesis.* Tense abdominal ascites can lead to an abdominal compartment syndrome and therefore impair renal function. If paracentesis is performed then ensure the patient receives adequate volume replacement for the ascites drained.

7 *Terlipressin* (Glypressin®): 0.5–1.0 mg intravenous four times daily. Should be considered in patients with HRS whose renal function fails to improve following adequate fluid resuscitation. Terlipressin is a synthetic analogue of vasopressin and causes peripheral and splanchnic vasoconstriction thereby ↓ splanchnic blood flow, ↓ portal hypertension and ↑ SVR. It is contraindicated in patients with coronary artery disease and peripheral vascular disease.

Haemofiltration/haemodialysis

If there is still no improvement in renal function or urine output despite the above steps then renal support should be considered early. Indications for haemofiltration include metabolic acidosis (pH <7.2) anuria, persistent hyperkalaemia and uraemia. Long-term dialysis may be required.

Renal biopsy

Rarely required but should be considered in patients with evidence of intrinsic renal disease. Can be performed percutaneously or via the transjugular route. Correction of coagulopathy may be required.

Joint liver–kidney transplantation

May be indicated in patients who have coexisting chronic liver and renal disease.

18 Cardiopulmonary complications

Hepatic hydrothorax
- Transudate pleural effusion
- Ascites from abdominal cavity passes into the pleural cavity

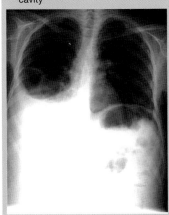

Cirrhosis and portal hypertension
- Splanchnic and peripheral vasodilatation
- Central hypovolaemia
- Arterial hypotension
- Increased cardiac output

Cirrhotic cardiomyopathy
- Blunted myocardial contractile response to stress
- Prolonged QT interval
- Features of congestive cardiac failure

Hepatopulmonary syndrome
- Dyspnoea
- Platypnea (dyspnoea exacerbated by standing)
- Orthodeoxia (hypoxaemia exacerbated by standing)
- Clubbing, cyanosis, spider naevi and telangactasia
- Contrast enhanced echocardiogram: microbubbles appear in left heart 3-6 cardiac cycles after injection entering right heart
- Intrapulmonary vascular dilatation

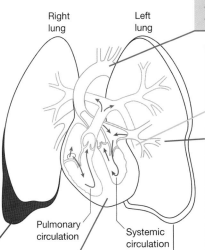

Right lung

Left lung

Pulmonary circulation

Systemic circulation

Pleura

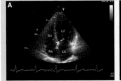
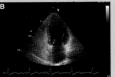
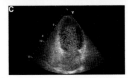

Source: *Goossens N, Joshi D & O'Grady J (2010).*

Contrast enhanced transsthoracic echocardiogram (A) four chamber view ; (B) appearance of microbubble contrast in the RA and RV, (C) delayed contrast appearing in the LA and LV four cycles after entering right cardiac chambers

Porto-pulmonary hypertension
- Progressive dyspnoea on exertion, syncope, chest pain and orthopnea
- Loud P2 and systolic murmur
- ECG: Right axis deviation, RBBB
- Pulmonary function tests: Decreased lung volumes, FVC, DLCO
- Right heart catheterisation: mPAP >25 mmHg, PCWP <15 mmHg

Haemodynamics of cirrhosis and cirrhotic cardiomyopathy

Cirrhosis and portal hypertension lead to splanchnic and peripheral vasodilatation, increased cardiac output and reduced tissue perfusion. Central hypovalaemia also occurs due to the redistribution of the effective circulating central blood volume. Baroreceptor activation and arterial hypotension leads to vasoconstriction via activation of the sympathetic nervous system. The haemodynamics of cirrhosis are very similar to that of sepsis. Autonomic dysfunction can also occur.

Cirrhotic cardiomyopathy is characterised by blunted myocardial contractile responsiveness to stress and/or diastolic relaxation with electrophysiological abnormalities such as prolongation of the QT interval in the absence of other known cardiac disease. Experimental studies have demonstrated reduced beta-adrenergic receptor signal transduction, nitric oxide over-production and altered transmembrane current and electromechanical coupling.

There is no specific therapy for cirrhotic cardiomyopathy. Management should be targeted towards congested heart failure with avoidance of vasodilators and angiotensin-converting enzyme (ACE) inhibitors. TIPS insertion may worsen cardiac function and should be avoided. Liver transplantation may result in improvement in cardiac dysfunction.

Porto-pulmonary hypertension

Porto-pulmonary hypertension (POPH) is characterised by pulmonary arterial hypertension (PAH) and portal hypertension (PHT) with or without advanced liver disease. Prevalence in liver transplant candidates varies between 5% and 9%. Risk factors include autoimmune hepatitis and female gender. Severity of POPH does not correlate with degree of liver impairment. The pathogenesis of POPH is incompletely understood. Proposed mechanisms include increased portal shunting resulting in increased exposure by the pulmonary vascular bed to vasoactive mediators which leads to pulmonary vasoconstriction and vascular remodelling.

Symptoms

Patients can present with symptoms of PAH or PHT. The most common symptom of PAH is progressive dyspnoea on exertion but others include syncope, chest pain and orthopnoea. Common clinical findings include an accentuated pulmonary component of the second heart sound, a systolic murmur consistent with tricuspid regurgitation and peripheral oedema.

Diagnosis

Other causes of PAH should be excluded. A transthoracic echocardiogram is a sensitive non-invasive screening tool to evaluate for PAH. Patients require right heart catheterisation to confirm PAH: mean pulmonary artery pressure (mPAP) >25 mmHg at rest; pulmonary capillary wedge pressure (PCWP) <15 mmHg.
- *ECG:* changes include right atrial and ventricular enlargement, right axis deviation and right bundle branch block (RBBB).
- *Imaging:* prominent or enlarged pulmonary arteries may be evident.
- *Lung function tests:* reduced lung volumes, forced vital capacity and carbon monoxide diffusing capacity (DLCO).

Treatment and prognosis

Without treatment, survival is poor. Medical management involves the use of vasomodulators and includes prostacyclin analogues (e.g. epoprostenol), endothelial receptor antagonists (e.g. bosentan) and phosphodiesterase-5-inhibitors (e.g. sildenafil). Response is assessed by serial echocardiography and measuring exercise tolerance using the 6-minute walk test. Liver transplantation remains an option but is contraindicated in patients with mPAP >50 mmHg.

Hepatopulmonary syndrome

Hepatopulmonary syndrome (HPS) is characterised by a triad of hepatic dysfunction, arterial oxygenation defect (with or without hypoxaemia) and intrapulmonary vascular dilatation (IPVD). HPS commonly occurs in cirrhosis but can occur in patients with non-cirrhotic portal hypertension. IPVD is integral in the pathogenesis of HPS and occurs secondary to nitric oxide release in response to bacterial translocation and increased pulmonary angiogenesis.

Symptoms

Dyspnoea is common. Platypnoea (dyspnoea exacerbated by standing) and orthodeoxia (hypoxaemia exacerbated by standing) can occur due to worsening ventilation–perfusion matching in the lung bases. Signs include clubbing, cyanosis, spider naevi and telangiectasia.

Diagnosis

HPS is diagnosed by demonstrating hypoxaemia and IPVD in the absence of intrinsic pulmonary disease. HPS can be catergorised as mild ($PaO_2 \geq 80$ mmHg), moderate (PaO_2 60–79 mmHg), severe (PaO_2 50–59 mmHg), and very severe ($PaO_2 < 50$ mmHg). IPVD is diagnosed using contrast-enhanced transthoracic echocardiography (agitated saline); microbubbles appear in the left heart 3–6 cardiac cycles after injection of contrast entering the right heart. Technetium-99-labelled macro-aggregated albumin can also be used with the appearance of technetium in the brain or spleen diagnostic of HPS.

Treatment and prognosis

Treatment options remain limited. Long-term oxygen is usually required. Liver transplantation is an effective option resulting in significant improvement in oxygenation and good 5-year survival rates (88%) in carefully selected individuals.

Hepatic hydrothorax

Hepatic hydrothorax is a complication of portal hypertension that is characterised by a transudate pleural effusion. It occurs in approximately 5–15% of cirrhotic patients. Ascites passes from the abdominal cavity into the pleural cavity due to a defect in the diaphragm, predominantly occurring in the right hemi-diaphragm. Symptoms include dyspnoea, cough and hypoxaemia. Management is as for ascites with dietary salt restriction with diuretics. Some patients may require drainage via the insertion of a chest drain but this should be avoided due to the high risk of complications. TIPS is indicated for refractory hepatic hydrothorax.

Hepatic encephalopathy

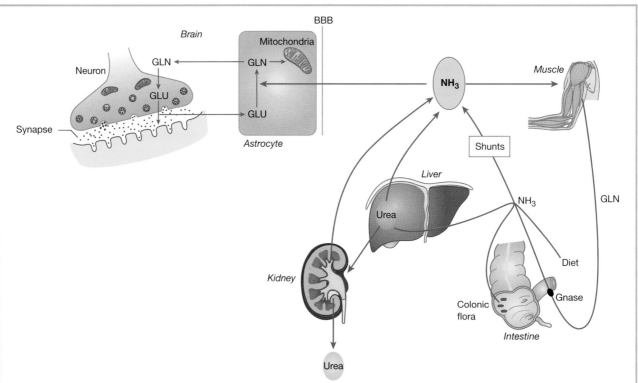

Figure 19-1 Pathogenesis of hepatic encephalopathy (HE). Source: *Garcia-Martinez R & Cordoba J (2011). Reproduced with permission of LWW.*

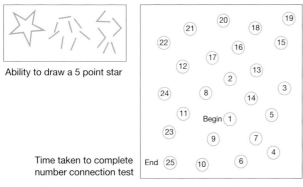

Ability to draw a 5 point star

Time taken to complete number connection test

Figure 19-2 Bedside psychometric tests for the diagnosis of HE.

Table 19-1 West Haven criteria for defining the severity of HE.

Grade 0	Minimal HE. No detectable changes in personality. Minimal changes in memory, concentration, intellectual function. Asterixis is absent
Grade 1	Short-term memory loss, euphoria, anxiety or lack of awareness. Reversed sleep-wake cycle
Grade 2	Lethargy, apathy, inappropriate behaviour, minimal disorientation and drowsiness. Asterixis is present
Grade 3	Somnolence to semi stupor but rousable, marked confusion and disorientation
Grade 4	Coma (unresponsive to painful stimuli)

Table 19-2 Medical treatments for HE.

Lactulose	Lactulose is the first line treatment for acute HE and for prophylaxis. It acts by acidifying the gut, which inhibits coliform bacteria converting urea into ammonia. In also has a cathartic effect, reducing colonic bacterial and urea load. Dosage: titrate to achieve >2 soft stool/day
Phosphate enemas	Particularly effective for HE >Grade 2, when patients are obtunded. Trying to administer lactulose in these situations is often problematic and usually futile
Rifaximin	Rifaximin is a non-absorbable antibiotic. In a recent large randomised study it has been shown to maintain remission from HE more effectively than placebo. Although widely used in Europe, North America and specialist centres in the UK, its use is currently not approved by the National Institute for Health and Care Excellence (NICE)
Probiotics	A recent systematic review has found probiotics to be an effective treatment for HE
Treatments no longer recommended for HE	High protein diets have not been found to exacerbate HE and dietary restriction is therefore not recommended. Neomycin has been shown to be an effective treatment for HE, but deafness can occur with long-term use and therefore routine use is no longer advocated. GABA antagonists (e.g. flumazenil) have not been shown to be consistently effective and in addition they have the potential to perpetuate seizures

Hepatology at a Glance, First Edition. Deepak Joshi, Geri Keane and Alison Brind.
© 2015 John Wiley & Sons, Ltd. Published 2015 by John Wiley & Sons, Ltd. Companion website: www.ataglanceseries.com/hepatology

Hepatic encephalopathy

Hepatic encephalopathy (HE) is defined as a 'spectrum of neuropsychiatric abnormalities in patients with liver dysfunction, after exclusion of other known brain disease'. It is characterised by changes in personality, intellectual impairment and drowsiness. HE can be subdivided into two main categories: overt and minimal. Overt HE is evident clinically, whereas minimal HE requires neuropsychological testing for confirmation.

Epidemiology

At any point in time, approximately one-third of patients with cirrhosis will have evidence of overt HE and nearly all others will have minimal HE. Patients with cirrhosis have an annual risk of developing overt HE of approximately 20%.

Type of HE (World Congress of Gastroenterology criteria)

A (Acute): acute and hyperacute liver failure;
B (Bypass): following TIPS or porto-systemic shunt surgery where the liver is bypassed. Liver disease may be absent;
C (Cirrhosis): cirrhosis with portal hypertension and portosystemic shunting. Can be further subdivided into:
  • episodic (precipitated, spontaneous, recurrent);
  • persistent (mild, severe or treatment-dependent); and
  • minimal encephalopathy.

Pathogenesis

The urea synthesis pathway is impaired in patients with liver disease and the brain (and muscle) acts as an alternative ammonia detoxification pathway. Astrocytes can convert ammonia into glutamine using the enzyme glutamine synthetase. However, if the brain receives a higher than normal ammonia load, then glutamine starts to accumulate in the astrocytes causing them to swell and malfunction. This leads to cerebral oedema and cytotoxic brain injury, which manifests as HE (Figure 19.1).

Common precipitants

• Non-compliance with HE therapy;
• Increased protein ingestion: gastrointestinal bleeding, excess dietary protein;
• Decreased ammonia excretion; constipation, renal failure;
• Electrolyte imbalance: hyponatraemia, hypovolaemia, hypokalaemia, alkalosis, hypoxia;
• Drugs (e.g. opiates, benzodiazepines, diuretics);
• Sepsis/inflammation;
• Paracentesis;
• Superimposed acute liver injury.

Grading of hepatic encephalopathy

HE is graded 0–4 using the West Haven criteria (Table 19.1). For > Grade 2 HE the Glasgow Coma Scale (GCS) is used in addition to report the level of depressed consciousness.

Diagnosis

HE is a clinical diagnosis and no single test is confirmatory.

Differential diagnosis:

• Intracranial lesions: subdural hematoma, intracranial bleeding, stroke, tumour, cerebral infection or post-ictal state;
• Metabolic encephalopathy: hypoglycaemia, diabetic ketoacidosis, hypoxia, hypercarbia, hyponatraemia, hypernatraemia, uraemia;
• Sepsis.
• Toxic encephalopathy: alcohol or drugs (e.g. sedatives).
• Wernicke's encephalopathy (acute thiamine deficiency)

History and clinical examination: Look for signs and symptoms of HE, such as asterixis and drowsiness as well as evidence of precipitating factors. Routine blood tests, blood cultures, urinalysis, chest X-ray and an ascitic tap should be considered in all patients. In those with a GCS of less than 8, the airway is potentially compromised and urgent assessment for ventilatory support by the anaesthetic or intensive care team is mandated.

Table 19.3

Investigations	Comments
Neuropsychological tests, e.g. 5-pointed star, number connection test (see Figure 19.2) or subtract serial 7's	These tests can be performed at the bed-side in patients with chronic liver disease and no overt HE. They demonstrate constructional apraxia which is diagnostic of minimal HE. Computer-based neuropsychometric tests are research tools which are currently being adapted for clinical use
Serum ammonia	60–90% of patients with HE will have an elevated serum ammonia. However, the test is neither sensitive nor specific for HE
CT head	A CT head in HE is typically normal except in Grade 3–4 HE when cerebral oedema may be present. However, it is an important test for ruling out other intracranial pathology
EEG	In HE EEGs may demonstrate high-amplitude low-frequency waves, triphasic waves or delta waves over the frontal lobes. However, these findings are non-specific and are often only present in Grade 3 or 4 HE. Can also differentiate HE from status epilepticus
MR head	Hyperintensity of the globus pallidus is sometimes seen on T1-weighted images
Visual evoked potentials	Unique patterns are demonstrated in HE but largely a research tool
Abdominal imaging	An abdominal US can identify precipitants (e.g. HCC). Multiphase contrast CT can be used to identify spontaneous portosystemic shunting (only indicated if high index of clinical suspicion)

Prognosis

HE in cirrhosis is considered to be a very poor prognostic sign. Following a hospital admission with overt HE, without liver transplantation 1-year survival is less than 50%. Many patients with HE will not be suitable for transplantation; however, early discussion with a transplant centre is always advised.

Management

• Identify and address precipitating factors (e.g. sepsis, gastrointestinal bleeding, drugs, constipation or hyponatremia).
• Diligent supportive care: correct hypovolaemia, electrolyte imbalances, sepsis and monitor for signs of cerebral oedema. In patients with HE without overt sepsis, have a low threshold for commencing broad-spectrum antibiotics. Ammonia excretion can be further improved through volume expansion or dialysis in patients with renal failure.
• Medical treatments (see Table 19.2).
• Liver transplantation.

Acute liver failure: 25% of hyper-acute and 9% of acute liver failure is associated with the development of cerebral oedema. Historically, the outlook for these patients was poor; however, survival has been significantly improved through the instigation of strategies to reduce cerebral oedema, intracranial hypertension and access to emergency liver transplantation. These patients should therefore be managed in specialist liver centres.

Acute liver failure

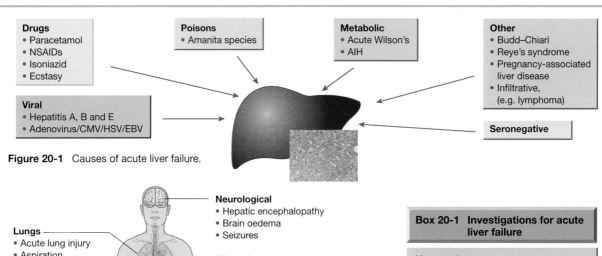

Drugs
• Paracetamol
• NSAIDs
• Isoniazid
• Ecstasy

Poisons
• Amanita species

Metabolic
• Acute Wilson's
• AIH

Other
• Budd–Chiari
• Reye's syndrome
• Pregnancy-associated
  liver disease
• Infiltrative,
  (e.g. lymphoma)

Viral
• Hepatitis A, B and E
• Adenovirus/CMV/HSV/EBV

Seronegative

Figure 20-1   Causes of acute liver failure.

Neurological
• Hepatic encephalopathy
• Brain oedema
• Seizures

Lungs
• Acute lung injury
• Aspiration

Adrenal
• Hypo-adrenalism

Cardiac
• Cardiovascular
  collapse
• Hypotension
• Tachycardia

Renal
• Acute kidney injury

Abdominal
• Ileus
• Pancreatitis
• Portal
  hypertension

Sepsis
• Bacterial
• Fungal

Bone marrow
• Low platelets

Figure 20-2   Clinical manifestations.

Box 20-1   Investigations for acute liver failure

Haematology
• Full blood count with blood film
• INR and clotting studies
• Haemolysis screen
• Pro-thrombotic screen*
• Bone marrow aspirate and trephine*

Biochemistry
• U and Es
• LFTs
• Arterial blood gases and arterial lactate
• Amylase
• Toxicology screen including
  paracetamol and salicylate levels
• Copper studies
• Serum urate*

Immunology
• Auto-antibodies
• Immunoglobulin profile

Virology/serology
• Heptitis A IgM
• Hepatitis B (sAg, sAb, IgM core
  Ab, viral load)
• Hepatitis C Ab and viral load
• Hepatitis E IgM and viral load
• CMV IgM and viral load
• HSV IgM and viral load
• Leptospira IgM

Imaging
• Doppler liver US
• CT with contrast

* When clinically indicated

Table 20-1   Classification.

	Hyperacute	**Acute**	**Subacute**
Time from jaundice to HE	0–7 days	1–4 weeks	4–12 weeks
Typical cause	Paracetamol	Hepatitis A, B and E	Drug induced (non-paracetamol)
Jaundice	Mild	Moderate	Severe
Coagulopathy	Severe	Moderate	Mild

Table 20-2   King's College criteria for transplantation.

Paracetamol-induced ALF	**Non-paracetamol induced ALF**
pH<7.3 (following volume resuscitation, irrespective of grade of HE) *or* Grade 3 or 4 HE Creatinine > 300 µmol/L INR >6.5 Arterial lactate >3.5 mmol/L at 4 h or >3 mmol/L at 12 h (following volume resuscitation)	INR > 6.5 *or* Any three of the following: • Etiology: seronegative hepatitis or drug induced • Age <10 or >40 years • Jaundice to encephalopathy >7 days • Bilirubin >300 µmol/L • INR >3.5

Hepatology at a Glance, First Edition. Deepak Joshi, Geri Keane and Alison Brind.
© 2015 John Wiley & Sons, Ltd. Published 2015 by John Wiley & Sons, Ltd. Companion website: www.ataglanceseries.com/hepatology

Acute liver failure

Acute liver failure (ALF) is characterised by the sudden loss of hepatic function due to hepatocyte necrosis resulting in hepatic encephalopathy (HE), jaundice and coagulopathy. ALF is rare, with an incidence of 1–6 cases/million/year in the Western world, and is associated with a high mortality. In the developing world, viral causes are more common than in the Western world where drug-induced liver injury predominates. Paracetamol (acetominophen) is commonly implicated in overdoses along with non-steroidal anti-inflammatory drugs (NSAIDs).

Definitions

ALF can be divided into three groups according to the onset of jaundice to the development of HE: hyperacute (0–7 days), acute (1–4 weeks) and subacute (4–12 weeks).

Clinical assessment and features

It is important to differentiate between ALF and decompensated CLD. A comprehensive history is essential, to elicit a history of CLD, previous episodes of self-harm, recent travel, pregnancy, 'high-risk' sexual behaviour or 'red-flag' malignancy symptoms. It is important to identify prescribed and non-prescribed medications. On examination, things to look for are signs of previous self-harm and signs of chronic liver disease (e.g. spider naevi and leuconychia). ALF is a multisystem disorder and therefore a thorough systemic review is essential.

Investigations

Serological tests for acute viral hepatitis should be performed if not clearly a paracetamol overdose. Patients testing negative should be assessed for other causes. Doppler US or cross-sectional imaging is required to ensure patency of the hepatic veins, look for evidence of chronic liver disease (e.g. signs of portal hypertension, nodular liver) and evidence of infiltrative malignancy. Liver biopsy is rarely helpful and high risk due to coagulopathy. If required, biopsy should be transjugular.

Management

General principles

Patients with ALF should be managed in a HDU or ITU setting with early discussion with the local transplant centre. Certain basic measures are routine.

Cardiovascular: Assessment of volume status. Intravascular volume depletion is common. ALF has similar characteristics to septic shock (i.e. low BP, peripheral vasodilatation, hyperdynamic circulation; ↑ heart rate, ↓ systemic vascular resistance, ↑ cardiac output). Central venous and arterial catheters may be required. The use of inotropic agents (e.g. norepinehrine) is common.

Respiratory: Is the patient able to protect their airway? Elective intubation is recommended in those with GCS <8 or severe agitation/confusion (i.e. grade 3 encepholopathy). Assessment of arterial blood gases. Respiratory complications include pneumonia, aspiration and acute lung injury.

Neurological: What is the GCS? Neurological dysfunction is common but can be subtle with rapid onset. Once the GCS is <8 the patient will have established brain oedema and will deteriorate rapidly. Once the patient has become agitated or develops grade 1 or 2 HE or GCS drops to 12, they should be immediately transferred to liver transplant centre. They should be intubated pre-transfer. Patients with high grade HE (>grade 3), young patients (<35 years) and those with a high serum ammonia level (>150 μmol/L) are at increased risk of developing cerebral oedema. Seizures are a poor prognostic sign. Intracranial monitoring may be required.

Renal and electrolytes: Renal dysfunction is common (>50%). Nephrotoxic drugs should not be given. Adequate volume resuscitation is required. The use of renal replacement therapy, if required, should be commenced early and is usually continuous veno-venous haemodialysis. Hypoglycaemia is common. ↑ Lactate reflects tissue hypoxaemia. Metabolic acidosis is common. Tight glucose control (6–10 mmol/L) is recommended. Avoid solutions that contain lactate (e.g. Hartmann's). Patients are often intravascular depleted.

Gastrointestinal: ALF is a hypercatabolic state and nutritional support is important.

Haematology: ↑ INR, ↓ platelets, ↓ fibrinogen. Correction of coagulopathy (fresh frozen plasma, platelets, cryoprecipitate) required only if there are signs of bleeding.

Infection: A comprehensive septic screen is recommended in all ALF patients due to the increased susceptibility to bacterial and fungal infections. Prophylactic antibiotics and antifungals are recommended. Universal precautions are integral to avoid nosocomial infections.

Specific measures:

Few specific therapies are available. *N*-acetylcysteine (NAC) is effective for paracetamol-induced hepatoxicity. For patients with non-paracetamol-induced ALF, NAC is also recommended. In cases of acute HBV or reactivation or flare of HBV, treatment with antivirals is recommended.

Role of liver transplantation

Liver transplantation remains the only definitive treatment for ALF as all other treatments are essentially supportive. The most widely used criteria are the King's College criteria which differentiate between paracetamol-induced and non-paracetamol-induced ALF. Survival post-liver transplantation for ALF patients has continued to improve and 1-year survival rates are in excess of 80%. Patients who are potential transplant candidates should be discussed and transferred early to their regional transplant centre.

Liver disease in pregnancy

Haemoglobin	↓ (from 2nd trimester)
White cell count	↑
Platelets	None
Packed cell volume	↓
PT/INR	None
ALP	↑ (bone and placenta)
Albumin	↓
ALT	None
GGT	None
Bilirubin	None
Alpha-fetoprotein	↑
Cholesterol	↑
Uric acid	↓

Figure 21-1 Changes in blood tests in pregnancy.

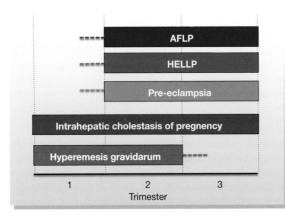

Figure 21-3 Timing of onset of pregnancy-related liver diseases.

HG	↑ Bili, ALT/AST
ICP	↑ Bili, ALT/AST, bile acids
Pre-eclampsia	↑ Bili, ALT/AST ↓ Platelets
HELLP	↑ ALT/AST, LDH, uric acid ↓ Platelets
AFLP	↑ Bili, ALT/AST, INR

Figure 21-4 Blood test abnormalities associated with pregnancy-related liver disease.

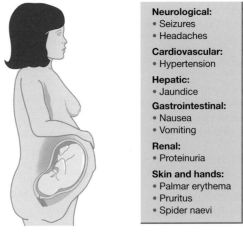

Neurological:
- Seizures
- Headaches

Cardiovascular:
- Hypertension

Hepatic:
- Jaundice

Gastrointestinal:
- Nausea
- Vomiting

Renal:
- Proteinuria

Skin and hands:
- Palmar erythema
- Pruritus
- Spider naevi

Figure 21-2 Signs and symptoms of liver disease in pregnancy.

Box 21-1   Classification of liver disease in pregnancy

Pregnancy-related liver diseases
- Hyperemesis gravidarum
- Intrahepatic cholestasis of pregnancy
- Pre-eclampsia and eclampsia
- HELLP syndrome
- Acute fatty liver of pregnancy

Pregnancy-unrelated liver diseases
Pre-existing liver diseases
- Cirrhosis and portal hypertension
- Hepatitits B and C
- Autoimmune liver disease
- Wilson's disease

Liver diseases co-incident with pregnancy
- Viral hepatitis
- Biliary disease
- Budd-Chiari syndrome
- Liver transplantation
- Drug-induced hepatotoxicity

HELLP = haemolysis, elevated liver enzymes and low platelets

Hepatology at a Glance, First Edition. Deepak Joshi, Geri Keane and Alison Brind.
© 2015 John Wiley & Sons, Ltd. Published 2015 by John Wiley & Sons, Ltd. Companion website: www.ataglanceseries.com/hepatology

During pregnancy, changes in maternal physiology and hormones are normal. Changes in liver biochemistry can also occur (see figure) but severe liver disease is rare. Classification of liver disease in pregnancy is shown in Box 21.1. Abdominal ultrasound and non-contrast MRI are safe in pregnancy. Liver biopsy is rarely required.

Pregnancy-related liver diseases
Hyperemesis gravidarum

Occurs in up to 2% of all pregnancies and in the first trimester. Onset is from week 4 and usually resolves by week 18. Hyperemesis gravidarum is characterised by intractable vomiting resulting in dehydration, ketosis and greater than 5% weight loss and non-specific rises in liver function tests. The cause remains unknown. Risk factors include high BMI, molar pregnancy, diabetes and multiple pregnancies. Treatment is supportive with intravenous hydration, antiemetics, vitamin supplementation especially thiamine, especially in severe cases. Relapse is common as is recurrence in subsequent pregnancies.

Intrahepatic cholestasis of pregnancy

This is defined as pruritus with elevated serum bile salts occurring in the second half of pregnancy, which resolves after delivery. A higher incidence of intrahepatic cholestasis of pregnancy (ICP) is observed in Scandinavia and South America. ICP can lead to placental insufficiency leading to fetal anoxia, prematurity, distress and stillbirth. Maternal morbidity is low. The cause is related to abnormal biliary transport across the canalicular membrane. Female sex hormones inhibit the bile salt export pump (BSEP) and mutations in *MDR3* are implicated. Pruritus, especially of the palms and soles, is the cardinal symptom, usually from week 25. Jaundice is uncommon. The key diagnostic test is a raised fasting serum bile acid (>10 µL/L). Ursodeoxycholic acid helps reduce pruritus, improves liver biochemistry and pregnancy outcome. ICP normally resolves after delivery. Recurrence in subsequent pregnancies is common.

Hypertension-related liver diseases in pregnancy
Pre-eclampsia and eclampsia

Pre-eclampsia affects 5–10% of pregnancies. It is characterised by hypertension and proteinuria (>300 mg/24 hours) after 20 weeks and/or within 48 hours of delivery. It is a multisystem disorder involving the kidneys, CNS, blood and the liver. Risk factors include extremes of maternal age, primiparity, hypertension, family history and previous history. Seizures differentiate eclampsia from pre-eclampsia. Placental ischaemia leading to endothelial dysfunction and coagulation activation has an important role. Symptoms include upper abdominal pain, nausea, vomiting and headache. Treatment involves BP control and intravenous magnesium sulfate may be given. Liver involvement suggests severe disease. Liver biochemistry usually normalises within 2 weeks of delivery.

HELLP (haemolysis, elevated liver enzymes, low platelets) syndrome

Some 5–10% of women with pre-eclampsia develop HELLP syndrome. HELLP is associated with a high infant mortality rate due to prematurity or secondary to maternal complications. It usually occurs in the second or third trimester but can also occur after delivery. Risk factors include advanced maternal age and multiparity. Clinical signs are similar to pre-eclampsia, with hypertension and proteinuria evident in up to 85% of patients.

Hepatic haematoma, infarction and rupture can occur and are diagnosed using CT or MRI. Raised aminotransferases (>1000 U/L), leucocytosis, pyrexia and anaemia are common findings. Blood transfusion, correction of coagulopathy and supportive care is recommended for contained haematomas. Haemodynamic instability suggests active bleeding and warrants surgical or radiological intervention.

Acute fatty liver of pregnancy

Acute fatty liver of pregnancy (AFLP) is rare. The majority present after 34 weeks. AFLP occurs due to abnormalities in β oxidation. Clinical features can include vomiting, hypoglycaemia, lactic acidosis, hyperammonaemia, hepatic encephalopathy and jaundice. Risk factors include twins and nulliparity. Raised aminotransferases, prothrombin time, uric acid and bilirubin are common. Microvesicular steatosis in hepatocytes occurs. Prompt delivery of the fetus is required; 60% are delivered within 24 hours. Liver transplantation maybe required in patients with hepatic failure.

Pre-existing liver diseases and pregnancy
Cirrhosis and portal hypertension

Pregnancy in cirrhotic women is rare due to decreased oestrogens, anovulation and amenorrhoea. Portal hypertension worsens due to increased blood volume and flow. Patients with varices have an increased risk of bleeding and therefore should undergo an OGD before pregnancy and at 20 weeks. The use of propranolol appears safe.

Liver diseases coincidental with pregnancy
Acute viral hepatitis

Worldwide the most prevalent viral cause of liver failure is hepatitis E virus infection. Infection is acquired usually in the second or third trimesters. There is a high maternal and fetal mortality rate. Treatment is supportive. Delivery does not appear to affect maternal outcome. HSV hepatitis is a rare disease but is more common in pregnancy. Mucocutaneuous lesions may be present. Survival is improved with intravenous aciclovir.

Other

Gallstones are more common in pregnancy in the second and third trimesters due to increased cholesterol secretion, decreased gallbladder motility and increased lithogenicity of bile. ERCP can be performed if required.

22 Indications for liver transplantation

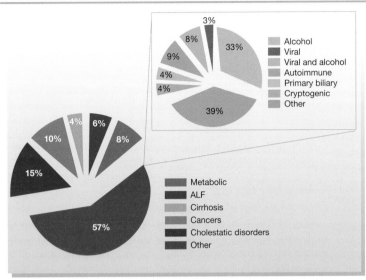

Alcohol — 33%
Viral — 39%
Viral and alcohol — 4%
Autoimmune — 4%
Primary biliary — 9%
Cryptogenic — 8%
Other — 3%

Metabolic
ALF — 15%
Cirrhosis — 57%
Cancers — 10%
Cholestatic disorders — 4%
Other — 6%, 8%

Figure 22-1 Cause of primary disease leading to liver transplantation.

Source: *Data taken from European Liver Transplant Registry.*

Box 22-1 Indications for liver transplantation: chronic liver disease

Cirrhosis with complications
- Synthetic dysfunction (MELD >15)

or
- Diuretic refractory ascites
- Recurrent hepatic encephalopathy
- Spontaneous bacterial peritonitis (SBP)

Hepatocellular carcinoma*

Other*
- Polycystic liver disease
- Inherited metabolic disorders
- Intractable itch for primary biliary cirrhosis
- Recurrent life-threatening biliary sepsis for primary sclerosing cholangitis
- Hepato-pulmonary syndrome
- Failed liver transplantation, i.e. primary non-function, hepatic artery thrombosis, chronic rejection, disease recurrence

* Irrespective of the MELD score

Box 22-1 Contraindications to liver transplantation

Absolute
- Active alcohol misuse or substance misuse
- Extrahepatic malignancy
- Multi organ failure
- Advanced cardiorespiratory disease
- Uncontrolled systemic sepsis
- Acquired immunodeficiency syndrome (AIDS)
- Severe psychiatric disease refractory to treatment

Relative
- Age >70 years
- Portal vein thrombosis with involvement of the mesenteric venous system
- Cumulative co-morbidity

Conventional technique

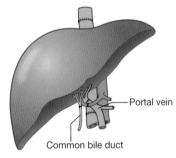

Portal vein
Common bile duct

Piggyback technique

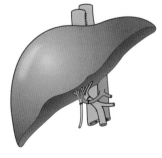

Split liver

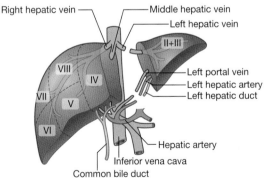

Right hepatic vein — Middle hepatic vein — Left hepatic vein
II+III
VIII
IV
Left portal vein
Left hepatic artery
Left hepatic duct
VII
V
VI
Hepatic artery
Inferior vena cava
Common bile duct

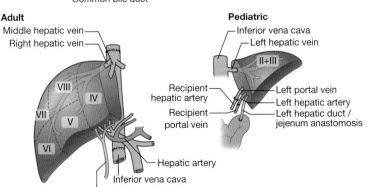

Adult
Middle hepatic vein
Right hepatic vein
VIII
IV
VII
V
VI
Hepatic artery
Inferior vena cava
Common bile duct

Pediatric
Inferior vena cava
Left hepatic vein
II+III
Recipient hepatic artery
Recipient portal vein
Left portal vein
Left hepatic artery
Left hepatic duct / jejenum anastomosis

Figure 22-2 Liver transplantation techniques.

Source: *Adapted from Zarrinpar, A. & Busuttil, R. Nat.Rev.Gastro.Hep. 10, 434–440 (2013).*

Hepatology at a Glance, First Edition. Deepak Joshi, Geri Keane and Alison Brind.
© 2015 John Wiley & Sons, Ltd. Published 2015 by John Wiley & Sons, Ltd. Companion website: www.ataglanceseries.com/hepatology

Liver transplantation

The first human liver transplant was performed in 1963. Since then outcomes have dramatically improved and liver transplantation (LT) is now an effective treatment for acute and chronic liver failure with 1 and 5 year survival rates greater than 90% and 70%, respectively. However, due to an increased number of transplant recipients – increased prevalence of chronic liver disease (CLD) and increased awareness of transplantation – there is a donor shortage. The result is an increased number of deaths on the waiting list.

Patient selection

When selecting a patient for LT a risk–benefit analysis must be undertaken taking into account the risks of surgery, immunosuppression and recurrent diseases weighed against the benefits of LT. Each patient therefore requires an individual assessment. Organs are allocated according to blood group. Timing of patient referral for LT can be difficult: too early, and the patient may not meet minimal listing criteria; too late, and the patient may be too sick to undergo LT.

Indications

LT for ALF is discussed in Chapter 40. Indications for LT with CLD (Box 22.1) are clinically based and supported by the Child–Pugh score and Model for End-stage Liver Disease (MELD) score in adults and the Paediatric End-stage Liver Disease (PELD) score in children <12 years.

Hepatocellular carcinoma

Criteria for LT are listed in Chapter 40.

Contraindications: absolute and relative

Absolute and relative contraindications are shown in Box 22.2.

HIV co-infection

HIV is no longer a contraindication to LT. HIV-positive patients require a CD4+ count >100 cells/mL and an undetectable HIV viral load. Caution is required in HIV–HCV co-infected cases due to accelerated recurrence rates of HCV post-LT.

Active alcohol use

Most transplant centres require a minimum period of 6 months abstinence. Alcoholic hepatitis remains a contraindication to LT in most centres but data from France have suggested a role for LT in selected patients who are unlikely to survive the 6-month period of sobriety.

Age

There is no upper age limit for LT. However, in older patients there is an increased likelihood of comorbidities especially malignancy and heart disease. Each patient therefore requires a thorough assessment.

Obesity

Data would suggest poorer outcomes in morbidly obese patients (BMI >40). Increased cardiovascular events have also been described in severely obese (BMI 35–40) patients. Patients with BMI >35 require a thorough dietetic assessment and enrolment in a weight reduction/exercise programme.

Patient assessment

Each patient requires a multidisciplinary holistic assessment to determine whether he/she is able to tolerate the stress of surgery, long-term immunosuppression and is committed to long-term LT care. The transplant assessment team includes a hepatologist, transplant surgeon, anaesthetist, intensive care physician, social worker, transplant nurse +/– substance misuse specialist.

Investigations include:
- *Blood tests:* FBC, U&Es, LFTs, coagulation profile, autoantibodies, iron studies, copper studies, α1-antitrypsin phenotype, CMV, EBV, HSV, varicella zoster virus, HIV, HAV-HDV serology, AFP;
- *Imaging:* CT/MRI to assess for HCC, patency of vasculature;
- *Endoscopy:* OGD, colonoscopy, MRCP (for patients with PSC).
- *Cardiovascular:* echocardiogram, ECG, coronary angiogram (for patients with >2 cardiac risk factors), cardiopulmonary exercise testing;
- *Pulmonary:* arterial blood gas (ABG), lung function tests, chest X-ray;
- *Psychosocial:* social work assessment, patient education, substance misuse assessment (if appropriate);
- *Other:* women also require PAP smear and mammogram (>35 years). All patients require testing for latent TB (IFN-γ testing).

Surgery

Types of donation

Organs can be used from donors after brain death (DBD) or after cardiac death (DCD). Donation from living donors is common in the Far East and from parents to their children. The left lateral lobe from the donor is usually used. A single adult liver can also be split and shared between two recipients, usually an adult and child. Auxillary LT involves the introduction of normal liver tissue but leaves the native liver *in situ*. It is rarely performed but can allow for the regeneration of the native liver especially in cases of ALF. Domino liver transplantation involves the use of a structurally normal liver but with a metabolic defect. Clinical manifestations of the metabolic defect in the recipient is usually delayed for 10–20 years.

Surgical procedure

The surgical operation usually takes 6 hours and blood loss is common. The hilar structures and the vena cava above and below the liver are dissected first. A 'piggy-back' implantation involves the confluence of the donor hepatic veins being anastomosed to the recipient vena cava. As the new liver is being implanted, splanchnic and vena caval circulation needs to be occluded. The order of anastomoses are as follows: (i) venous (intrahepatic vena cava then portal vein); (ii) arterial (hepatic artery to hepatic artery) and then; (iii) biliary (bile duct to bile duct or Roux-en-Y choledochojejunostomy).

Postoperative care

Patients are normally managed for 24–48 hours in an intensive care setting. A liver US scan is required within 24 hours to ensure patency of the hepatic artery. A steady fall in serum transaminases (AST/ALT), bilirubin and INR should be seen every 12 hours.

23 Drug-induced liver injury

Age

Toxicity is more common at the extremes of age, partly because of increased chances of drug interactions in the elderly and significant co-morbidities. There are also classical age-dependent disorders (e.g. Reye's syndrome – childhood aspirin-induced microvesicular steatosis)

Gender

Females may be more susceptible to flucloxacillin, methyldopa and nitrofurantoin, and males to azathioprine and co-amoxiclav cholestatic hepatitis

Nutritional state

Depletion of glutathione by fasting, pregnancy or alcohol increases the risks of paracetamol and intravenous tetracycline toxicity in pregnancy

Chronic alcohol abuse

Affects toxicity by enzyme induction and common pathways of injury such as steatohepatitis (increased susceptibility to methotrexate)

Obesity and diabetes

Affect susceptibility to steatosis

Systemic disease

May predispose to drug damage – particularly in halothane hepatitis

Genetic variants in metabolising enzymes

Conjugating enzymes
- Functional or genetic changes in UDP-glucuronosyltransferases (UGT) sulfotransferases and glutathione–S-transferases affect toxicity
- Gilbert's syndrome caused by mutation in *UGT1A1* may increase susceptibility to irinotecan DILI
- Inactive *N*-acetyltransferase increases susceptibility to sulphonamide and hydralazine DILI
- Deficiency of functional sulfoxidation susceptibility to chlorpromazine DILI

Oxidation
- There are many common polymorphysms of cytochrome P450 (CYP) which are important in oxidation of many drugs. Not surprisingly, functional polymorphisms are probably important in susceptibility to many drugs (e.g. P4502D6 and P4502C19 to perhexilene and hydralazine DILI)

Biliary transport
- Genetic variation in biliary transport proteins will affect susceptibility to cholestatic reactions

Immune response
- Immune reactions may be influenced by HLA polymorphisms

Flucloxacillin and coamoxiclav DILI are associated with HLA haplotype

HLA haplotype (*HLA-DRB1*1501-HLA-DQB1*0602-HLA-DRB5*0101-HLADQA1*0102*) and lumiracoxib-induced hepatotoxicity

In addition, certain DILI with immune hepatitis features is associated with antibodies to certain P450 enzymes (P5402C9 and 1A2)

Injury pattern	Common causative drugs
Hepatocellular	NSAIDs, leflunamide, anaesthetic drugs eg halothane, rifampicin, ketoconazole, antiretrovirals, ecstasy
Acute cholestatic hepatitis	Co-amoxiclav, flucloxacillin, NSAIDs, carbamezipine, allopurinol, oesotrogens and anabolic steriods
Chronic cholestasis and ductopenia	Carbamazepine, co-amoxiclav, co-trimoxazole, erythromycin, flucloxacillin, methyltestosterone, phenytoin, azathioprine, cyclosporine (pure cholestasis)
Drug-induced autoimmune hepatitis	Infliximab, diclofenac, indomethacin, minocycline, nitrofurantoin, pegylated interferon
Granulomatous hepatitis	Allopurinol, carbamazapine, isoniazid, sulphfonylureas
Steatosis	
• Microvesicular	Tetracycline, aspirin, valproate, nucleoside analogues
• Macrovesicular	Methotrexate, amiodarone, nifedipine, tamoxifen corticosteroids, methotrexate
Vascular lesions Hepatic vein thrombosis/ veno-occlusive disease	Azathioprine, dacarbazine, combination chemotherapy (haematological), oral contraceptives
Nodular regenerative hyperplasia, veno-occlusive disease, peliosis hepatic, sinusoidal dilatation	Anabolic and contraceptive steroids, toxic oil, pyrrolidine alkaloids – bush tree, azathioprine, chemotherapy (haematological) vitamin A
Hepatocellular carcinoma and adenoma	Anabolic and contraceptive steroids

Definitions

An **adverse drug reaction (ADR)** is defined as any response to a drug that is noxious, is unintended and occurs at doses normally used in humans for the prophylaxis, diagnosis or therapy of disease.

An **idiosyncratic drug-induced liver injury (DILI)** is an ADR that is unexpected on the basis of the pharmacological action of the drug administered.

Epidemiology

The estimated annual incidence rate of DILI in the UK is 14 per 100 000. DILI accounts for disproportionate number of serious or fatal ADRs: 3.5–9.5% of all drug reactions but 14.7% of serious or fatal ADRs. Drugs are thought to be responsible for 2–6% of cases of jaundice, 10% of 'acute hepatitis' and 10–20% of acute liver failure. Up to 6% of chronic hepatitis may be drug induced. DILI is thought to be an important cause of cholestasis, but this has been not quantified. Drugs may also contribute to the aetiology of up to 1% of liver tumours.

Drugs are extensively tested before becoming available for clinical use so it is rare that ADRs are seen (1 in 10 000–100 000) in licensed drugs. Their recognition depends on vigilance and post-market surveillance (e.g. Yellow Card reporting). Several drugs have been withdrawn post-licensing because of the occurrence of DILI (e.g. troglitazone, ketoconazole and lumiracoxib). DILI can occur with OTC drugs, recreational drugs and herbal remedies.

Mechanisms

In the majority of cases, liver injury occurs due to the direct toxic effect of the drug (>60%) or its metabolite. In other cases, injury results from an immunological reaction to either the drug or the active metabolite formed by bioactivation. DILI can be idiosyncratic or dose dependent.

Risk factors

DILI is more prevalent at the extremes of age, in those who are malnourished or who have existing liver disease. Further drug-specific risk factors are outlined in the table. The manifestation of DILI is dependent on environmental triggers in those with a genetic susceptibility. In the future, genetic profiling may be used to assess the risk of DILI versus the potential benefit of a drug.

Diagnosis

Adverse hepatic reactions can mimic a wide spectrum of hepato-biliary diseases. Early recognition and prompt withdrawal of the drug is essential. Failure to detect hepatotoxicity at an early stage may be fatal and an inaccurate diagnosis may lead to the inappropriate withdrawal of an effective medication.

Diagnosis depends on a high level of suspicion and systematic assessment. DILI may be symptomatic or asymptomatic and be detected by abnormal liver blood tests checked routinely or during drug monitoring. Patterns of DILI and commonly implicated drugs are listed. A drug usually causes a particular pattern of liver injury but a few drugs cause various patterns – there are some classic patterns. DILI can be defined as:

5× ULN ALT; or
>2× ULN ALP; or
>3× ULN ALT and 2× ULN bilirubin.

There is usually a temporal relationship between manifestation of injury and therapy. In hepatocellular or cholestatic hepatitis time from drug institution to injury is 1 day to 8 weeks (or 1 day on rechallenge) but DILI may occur after a drug has been discontinued or occur after a significant duration of therapy. Steatohepatitis or vascular injury have a more insidious onset. On some occasions tolerance to DILI occurs and abnormal liver blood tests and injury resolve despite ongoing therapy (e.g. statin therapy).

Assessment of suspected DILI

- Drug with established history of DILI;
- Indication for use of drug;
- Dates of treatment;
- Initial biochemical abnormality and trends in liver biochemistry;
- Associated systemic features and timing of onset – fever, rash, eosinophilia, cytopenia, arthralgia;
- Exclusion of other potential causes.

These factors form part of the DILI diagnostic score. In equivocal cases this can be used or a more comprhensive scoring system such as the Roussel Uclaf Causality Assessment (RUCAM).

Re-challenge may occasionally be used to aid diagnosis. Re-challenges should be performed with great caution in immune-mediated DILI. Liver biopsy is rarely required unless there is an atypical presentation or need to assess degree of chronic damage and prognosis (e.g. methotrexate).

Dress syndrome

Dress syndrome is a drug rash with eosinophilia and systemic symptoms. Three of the following clinical features are necessary for diagnosis: fever, exanthema, eosinophilia, atypical circulating lymphocytes, lymphadenopathy and hepatitis. Idiosyncratic reaction occurs most commonly after exposure to drugs such as allopurinol, sulfonamides and aromatic anticonvulsants such as phenytoin, phenobarbital and carbamazepine.

24 Focal liver lesions

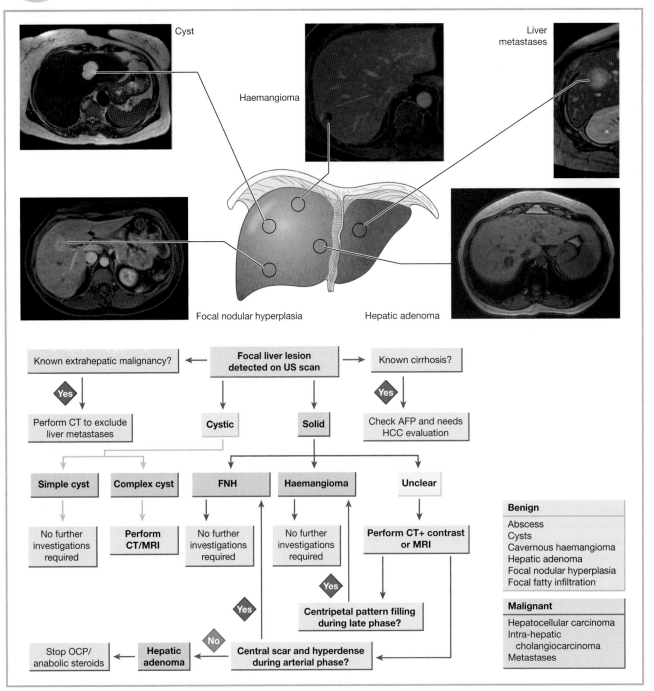

Cyst

Haemangioma

Liver metastases

Focal nodular hyperplasia

Hepatic adenoma

Benign
Abscess
Cysts
Cavernous haemangioma
Hepatic adenoma
Focal nodular hyperplasia
Focal fatty infiltration

Malignant
Hepatocellular carcinoma
Intra-hepatic cholangiocarcinoma
Metastases

Flow chart:

Focal liver lesion detected on US scan

- Known extrahepatic malignancy? → **Yes** → Perform CT to exclude liver metastases
- Known cirrhosis? → **Yes** → Check AFP and needs HCC evaluation
- Cystic
  - Simple cyst → No further investigations required
  - Complex cyst → **Perform CT/MRI**
- Solid
  - FNH → No further investigations required
  - Haemangioma → No further investigations required
  - Unclear → Perform CT+ contrast or MRI → Centripetal pattern filling during late phase? → **Yes** → Haemangioma
    - Central scar and hyperdense during arterial phase? → **Yes** → FNH
    - → **No** → Hepatic adenoma → Stop OCP/anabolic steroids

Hepatology at a Glance, First Edition. Deepak Joshi, Geri Keane and Alison Brind.
© 2015 John Wiley & Sons, Ltd. Published 2015 by John Wiley & Sons, Ltd. Companion website: www.ataglanceseries.com/hepatology

The discovery of an incidental focal liver lesion is common. These can be asymptomatic or symptomatic, occurring in the absence or presence of liver disease. Many are asymptomatic and are incidental findings on liver imaging. It is important to assess for chronic liver disease or evidence of extrahepatic malignancy. Imaging modalities including ultrasound (US), computed tomography (CT) and magnetic resonance imaging (MRI) can usually differentiate between the causes. Fine needle aspiration (FNA) or biopsy are sometimes required in cases where imaging is not diagnostic.

Benign lesions

Abscess

Liver abscesses can be pyogenic, arising from local, distal infection or due to amoebiasis. Patients present with right upper quadrant pain and evidence of sepsis (↑ WCC, pyrexia). Amoebic liver abscesses are usually solitary and occur in the right lobe. Cysts secondary to hydatid infection should be considered.

Imaging: On US and CT scans, pyogenic abscesses can be solitary or multiple with poorly defined irregular margins with areas of coarse debris or fluid–debris levels.

Management: Antibiotics ± drainage.

Cysts

Simple cysts are common, affecting nearly 3% of the general population. Cysts can single or multiple and can occur as part of systemic disease (e.g. polycystic kidney disease). If large, they can become symptomatic due to a mass pressure effect.

Imaging: On US, cysts are anechoic and have a well-defined thin wall. Complex cysts may demonstrate internal septae and irregular thickening of the walls. In complex cysts, further evaluation with CT is often required as malignant lesions cannot be confidently excluded.

Management: Small cysts do not require any treatment. Symptomatic cysts may require US or CT guided drainage. Rarely, surgery is required for larger cysts.

Hepatic haemangioma

More common in women, this is the most common benign hepatic lesion. Patients are normally asymptomatic and may have evidence of haemangiomas in other sites (e.g. lung, skin or brain). The risk of rupture is low given that it is a low-pressured system. Thrombosis can occur within cavernous haemangiomas. Liver biochemistry is often normal.

Imaging: On US, a peripheral solitary uniform echogenic mass is seen. The border is well demarcated with no peripheral halo. There is minimal flow to the liver on Doppler imaging. CT + contrast demonstrates peripheral nodular enhancement in the early phase and pooling of contrast in the late phase.

Management: No further investigation required. Symptomatic larger lesions rarely may require resection.

Focal nodular hyperplasia

Also known as hepatic hamartoma, focal nodular hyperplasia (FNH) is characterised by a nodular hyperplastic hepatic lesion. An anomalous arterial supply within these regenerative nodules is key to the pathogenesis. Also more common in women (ratio 10 : 1), up to 3% of population are affected. There can be an association with use of the oral contraceptive pill (OCP) but no proven pathogenic role. Can be associated with abnormal LFTs (↑ GGT). Can be single or multiple but usually <5 cm diameter.

Imaging: A well-demarcated border with no true capsule is noted on US. The characteristic finding is a hypoechoic central scar. A 'spoke-wheel' pattern is noted on Doppler studies. A CT during the arterial phase demonstrates the characteristic punctuate enhancement in the central scar in a hyperdense lesion. MR can also demonstrate the central scar and may be more appropriate in younger patients.

Management: No further investigations required if diagnosis is secure. FNH is not a contraindication to hormone replacement therapy, OCP or pregnancy.

Hepatic adenoma

Hepatic adenoma is a benign proliferation of hepatocytes, occurring in a non-cirrhotic liver. It is associated with the use of the OCP and can occur in men who have used anabolic steroids. Tends to occur in the right lobe.

Imaging: A hyper-echoic solitary lesion, although multiple lesions can occur especially in patients with glycogen storage diseases. A central hypo-echoic region representing haemorrhage may also be seen on US because of an increased risk of bleeding. Findings on CT and MRI are non-specific and often requires biopsy for definitive diagnosis. Minimal Kupffer cells are present, and therefore a focal defect is noted on scintigraphy.

Management: Stop OCP and anabolic steroids. Surgical resection to be considered due to the risk of malignant transformation into HCC and risk of rupture. Size can increase in pregnancy.

Focal fatty infiltration or sparing

Fat can accumulate focally with areas of focal infiltration or sparing too. It is common in patients with diabetes, hyperlipidaemia, obesity, those who drink alcohol or take steroids.

Imaging: On US, fat is hyper-echoic. On CT, fat has low attenuation. There is increased signal on T1-weighted images using MRI.

Management: No specific treatment required (see Chapter 27).

Malignant lesions

Metastases represent the most common malignant tumours of the liver in the Western world. Lesions are often multiple and can involve both lobes. It is important to identify the primary malignancy and exclude primary liver malignancy (see Chapter 40).

Imaging: Adenocarcinomas (stomach, pancreas and colon) are hypo-echoic on US scan and appear as low attenuation lesions in the portal venous phase on CT/MRI and are hypovascular. Metastases from breast, thyroid, renal cell carcinoma and melanoma are hypervascular and enhanced in the arterial phase on CT. MRI is particular good at identifying vascular involvement.

Management: Depends on underlying primary. A multidisciplinary approach is recommended.

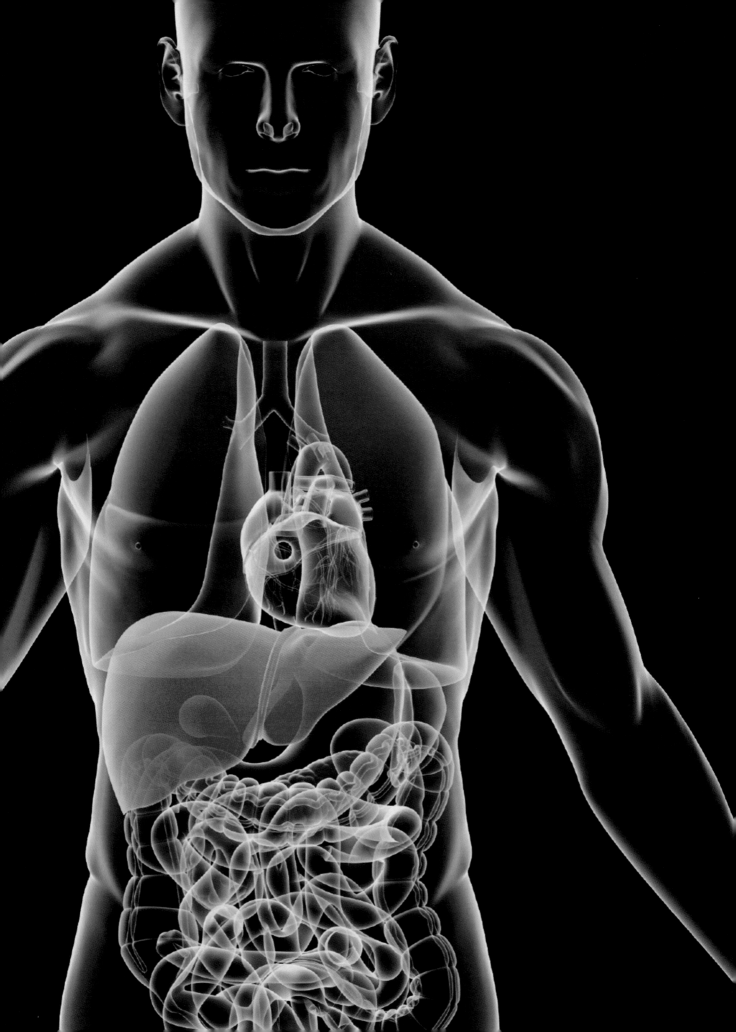

Diseases

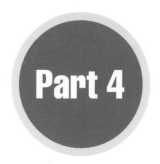

Part 4

Chapters

Visit the companion website at
www.ataglanceseries.com/hepatology
to test yourself on these topics

25 Alcohol-related liver disease

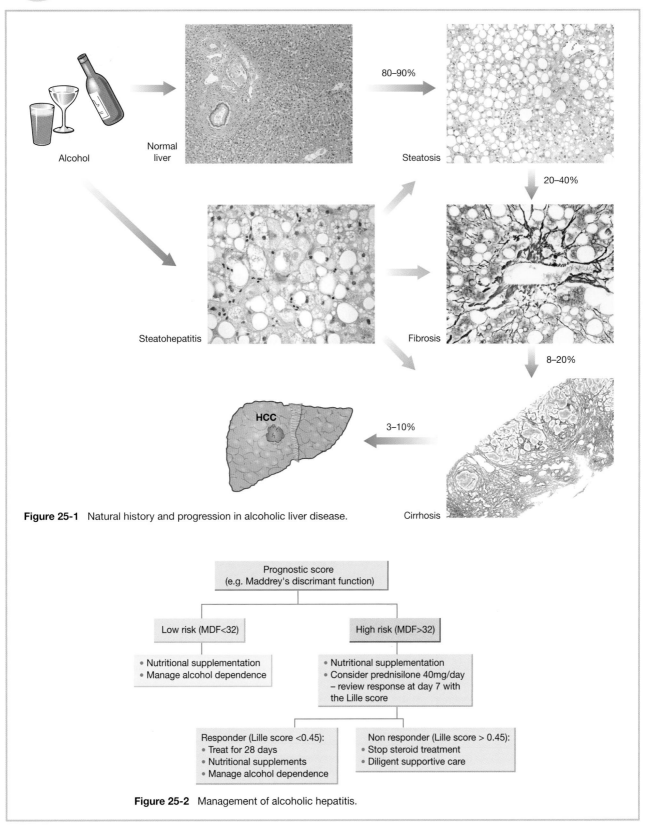

Figure 25-1 Natural history and progression in alcoholic liver disease.

Alcohol → Normal liver → 80–90% → Steatosis → 20–40% → Fibrosis → 8–20% → Cirrhosis → 3–10% → HCC

Steatohepatitis

Figure 25-2 Management of alcoholic hepatitis.

Prognostic score
(e.g. Maddrey's discrimant function)

Low risk (MDF<32)
- Nutritional supplementation
- Manage alcohol dependence

High risk (MDF>32)
- Nutritional supplementation
- Consider prednisilone 40mg/day
  – review response at day 7 with the Lille score

Responder (Lille score <0.45):
- Treat for 28 days
- Nutritional supplements
- Manage alcohol dependence

Non responder (Lille score > 0.45):
- Stop steroid treatment
- Diligent supportive care

Hepatology at a Glance, First Edition. Deepak Joshi, Geri Keane and Alison Brind.
© 2015 John Wiley & Sons, Ltd. Published 2015 by John Wiley & Sons, Ltd. Companion website: www.ataglanceseries.com/hepatology

In England and Wales, alcohol consumption has doubled since the mid-1950s and more than one-third of the population are thought to exceed recommended consumption limits.

Pathogenesis

The liver metabolises more than 90% of all ingested alcohol and in excess consumption it is this process that is primarily responsible for the subsequent liver injury. Within the liver there are two main pathways for the metabolism of alcohol: alcohol dehydrogenase and cytochrome P-450 (CYP) 2E1. Both pathways convert alcohol to acetaldehyde, which is fundamental in alcohol-mediated liver injury. In addition, acetetaldehyde activates the hepatic stellate cells, which produce cytokines including TNF-α, which increase the production of reactive oxygen species, causing inflammation, hepatocyte necrosis, extracellular matrix remodelling and fibrogenesis. Chronic alcohol consumption also inhibits gluconeogenesis and causes triglyceride accumulates within the hepatocytes.

Alcohol-related liver diseases

ALD can manifest as fatty liver disease, alcoholic hepatitis or cirrhosis. It is not certain that these diseases represent a continuum, as significant overlap exists between these groups. Histologically, ALD can look identical to NAFLD or drug toxicity so medical history and documentation of current and historical alcohol consumption is critical.

Steatosis

Alcohol-related fatty liver is mostly asymptomatic and often diagnosed as a result of the discovery of abnormal liver biochemistry in high alcohol consumers. An ultrasound of the liver will demonstrate fatty infiltration. A biopsy is rarely necessary unless the aetiology or stage of disease is unclear. However, if undertaken it will demonstrate macrovesicular fat accumulating in the hepatocytes, predominantly in the central and mid-zonal areas. Fatty liver is a reversible condition with cessation of hazardous drinking; however, if patients continue to consume alcohol its presence increases the likelihood of progression to cirrhosis.

Steatohepatitis

The classic histological features of steatohepatitis are the presence of inflammation and necrosis, demonstrated by the presence of ballooning hepatocytes (which can cause compression of the sinusoid and reversible portal hypertension), necroinflammation, Mallory bodies, neutrophil infiltrate and megamitochrondria. Steatohepatitis is triggered by continued significant alcohol consumption or an alcohol binge. Severe steatohepatitis manifests clinically as alcoholic hepatitis. Mild forms may be asymptomatic. There is significant likelihood that steatohepatitis will progress to cirrhosis without abstinence.

Cirrhosis

Cirrhosis can present with decompensation or be an incidental finding on imaging. A liver biopsy will show pericentral and perivenular zone fibrosis (chicken wire fibrosis) prior to cirrhosis. Established cirrhosis is irreversible. Patients with decompensation have a poor prognosis. However, most patients will recompensate with abstinence. Long-term, patients remain at risk of portal hypertension, oesophageal varices and HCC and therefore require regular surveillance. If patients deteriorate despite abstinence they should be considered for transplant assessment.

Hepatocellular carcinoma

In the UK in 2010 approximately 9% of HCCs were attributed to alcohol consumption. Chronic alcohol use of greater than 80 g/day for more than 10 years increases the risk of HCC fivefold, compared to the general population. Additional risk factors for HCC (see Chapter 40) further increase the risk. Typically, HCCs develop in cirrhotic livers. The pathogenesis of alcohol-induced HCC is incompletely understood, but may be triggered by mechanisms such as chromosomal loss, oxidative stress altered DNA methylation and genetic susceptibility.

Alcoholic hepatitis

Alcoholic hepatitis is a clinical diagnosis. Patients present with jaundice, malaise, abdominal pain, diarrhoea, vomiting, anorexia and confusion. Hepatomegaly, ascites, encephalopathy and malnutrition are common findings on examination.

Management of alcoholic hepatitis

The treatment of alcoholic hepatitis primarily involves the management of complications such as encephalopathy, sepsis, malnutrition or portal hypertension. Further management is dependent on severity (see algorithm), which is assessed using prognostic scores (e.g. Maddrey's discriminate function, DF, or the Glasgow Hepatitis Score, GHS).

$$DF = 4.6\,(PT - normal\ PT\ in\ seconds) + bilirubin$$

Steroids: Corticosteroids (40 mg prednisolone) can be considered when the DF is >32. Use of corticosteroids is associated with a survival benefit of 20–50%, in the absence of uncontrolled sepsis or variceal bleeding. Response is monitored using the Lille score. A fall in bilirubin after 1 week is associated with a good prognosis.

$$R = 3.19 - 0.101 \times [age(years)] + 0.147 \times [albumin\ on\ day\ 0(g/L)]$$
$$+ 0.0165 \times [evolution\ in\ bilirubin\ level\ (\mu mol / L)] -$$
$$0.206 \times renal\ insufficiency - 0.0065 \times$$
$$[bilirubin\ on\ day\ 0(mol/L)] - 0.0096 \times [PT\ (seconds)]$$
$$Lille\ score = exp(-R)/[1 + exp(-R)]$$

Note: Renal insufficiency = 1 if present and 0 if absent. Evolution in billirubin level is bilirubin on day 0 minus that on day 7.

Pentoxifylline (400 mg three times daily): Recommended for severe alcoholic hepatitis, especially when there are contraindications to corticosteroid use (ASSLD) or, if sepsis, precludes steroid use (EASL). A recent Cochrane review showed pentoxyfylline can reduce mortality in severe alcoholic hepatitis.

Nutrition: Malnutrition correlates strongly with short and long-term mortality in alcoholic hepatitis. Enteral nutrition can be as effective as steroids in the treatment of severe alcoholic hepatitis (see Chapter 49).

Transplantation: A 6-month abstinence from alcohol is typically required before patients with any alcohol-related liver disease are considered for liver transplantation. However, emerging evidence suggests good outcomes can be achieved in carefully selected patients with alcoholic hepatitis, but it remains a controversial indication.

26 Management of alcohol misuse

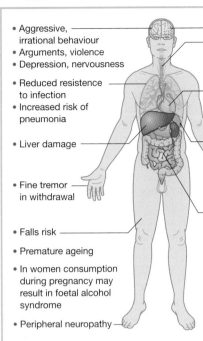

- Aggressive, irrational behaviour
- Arguments, violence
- Depression, nervousness

- Reduced resistence to infection
- Increased risk of pneumonia

- Liver damage

- Fine tremor in withdrawal

- Falls risk

- Premature ageing

- In women consumption during pregnancy may result in foetal alcohol syndrome

- Peripheral neuropathy

- Memory loss
- Increased risk of cancer particularly of the throat, mouth, oesophagus, liver and breast
- Heart failure, arrhythmias
- Anaemia
- Impaired blood clotting
- Breast cancer
- Pancreatitis

- Gastrointestinal haemorrhage, peptic ulcer disease, vitamin deficiency and malnutrition

Figure 26-1 Complications of alcohol misuse.

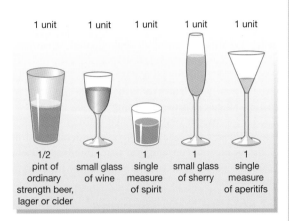

1 unit	1 unit	1 unit	1 unit	1 unit
1/2 pint of ordinary strength beer, lager or cider	1 small glass of wine	1 single measure of spirit	1 small glass of sherry	1 single measure of aperitifs

Figure 26-2 Drinks and units.
Each drink represents one alcohol unit which contains 10 mL pure alcohol

The Alcohol Use Disorders Identification Test: Self-Report Version

PATIENT: Because alcohol use can affect your health and can interfere with certain medications and treatments, it is important that we ask some questions about your use of alcohol. Your answers will remain confidential so please be honest.

Place an X in one box that best describes your answer to each question

Table 26.1 AUDIT questionnaire. Source: *Babor TF et al. (2001). Reproduced with permission of WHO.*

Questions	0	1	2	3	4
1. How often do you have a drink containing alcohol?	Never	Monthly or less	2-4 times a month	2-3 times a week	4 or more times a week
2. How many drinks containing alcohol do you have on a typical day when you are drinking?	1 or 2	3 or 4	5 or 6	7 or 9	10 or more
3. How often do you have six or more drinks on one occasion?	Never	Less than monthly	Monthly	Weekly	Daily or almost daily
4. How often during the last year have you found that you were not able to stop drinking once you had started?	Never	Less than monthly	Monthly	Weekly	Daily or almost daily
5. How often during the last year have you failed to do what was normally expected of you because of drinking?	Never	Less than monthly	Monthly	Weekly	Daily or almost daily
6. How often during the last year have you needed a first drink in the morning to get yourself going after a heavy drinking session?	Never	Less than monthly	Monthly	Weekly	Daily or almost daily
7. How often during the last year have you had a feeling of guilt or remorse after drinking?	Never	Less than monthly	Monthly	Weekly	Daily or almost daily
8. How often during the last year have you been unable to re-member what happened the night before because of your drinking?	Never	Less than monthly	Monthly	Weekly	Daily or almost daily
9. Have you or someone else been injured because of your drinking?	No		Yes, but not in the last year		Yes during the last year
10. Has a relative, friend, doctor or other health care worker been concerned about your drinking or suggested you cut down?	No		Yes, but not in the last year		Yes, during the last year

Hepatology at a Glance, First Edition. Deepak Joshi, Geri Keane and Alison Brind.

Harmful drinking is defined as a pattern of alcohol consumption that leads to health or social problems, which are directly related to alcohol. This includes psychological problems such as depression, alcohol-related accidents or physical illnesses such as liver disease, pancreatitis, neuropathy, dementia, Wernicke–Korsakoff syndrome, cardiomyopathy and certain types of cancer. In the UK, one-quarter of the population are defined as harmful drinkers and more than 1 million hospital admissions every year are attributed to alcohol.

Alcohol dependence is characterised by craving, tolerance, preoccupation with alcohol and continued drinking in spite of resultant physical, psychological or social harm. Alcohol dependence affects 4% of people aged between 16 and 65 in England.

Recommended alcohol consumption limits

The Department of Health recommend weekly alcohol consumption should not exceed 21 units for men and 14 units for women (Figure 26.2).

Screening for alcohol misuse

Individuals presenting with conditions that may be a consequence of alcohol misuse should be screened for harmful consumption using the Alcohol Use Disorders Identification Test (AUDIT) (Table 26.1). Harmful drinking is defined as an AUDIT score of >15. High AUDIT scores (>20) suggest alcohol dependency.

Assessment

- Alcohol consumption including historical and recent patterns of drinking. Additional information, from family members or carers is often useful.
- Alcohol dependency is assessed using the Severity of Alcohol Dependence Questionnaire (SADQ).
- Alcohol-related physical health problems (Figure 26.1).
- Psychiatric and social problems.
- Other drug misuse, including OTC medication.
- Cognitive function (e.g. Mini Mental State Examination, MMSE).
- Readiness for change.

Management

Abstinence is an important goal for most people with alcohol dependence and harmful drinking. However, many find this challenging and moving to moderate level consumption may be all that is acceptable.

Hazardous and harmful drinking (AUDIT >15)

Those with hazardous or harmful drinking require brief interventions with advice to encourage abstinence. Brief interventions can be undertaken by any health care professional. The key elements are helping people to recognise problems related to their drinking and encourage change. The FRAMES acronym provides a useful method for clinicians to structure the intervention interview:

- *Feedback:* about personal risk or impairment.
- *Responsibility:* emphasis on personal responsibility for change.
- *Advice:* to cut down or abstain if indicated because of severe dependence or harm.
- *Menu:* of alternative options for changing drinking behaviour. Set targets and achievable intermediate goals jointly with the patient.
- *Empathic interviewing:* listening reflectively without cajoling or confronting the patient. Explore how they see themselves and their reasons for change.
- *Self-efficacy:* adopt an interviewing style that enhances people's belief in their ability to change.

Dependent drinking

Those with dependent drinking should be referred to addiction services. They are likely to require withdrawal management as well as specialised interventions such as individual psychological intervention or self-help groups (e.g. Alcoholics Anonymous), counselling, cognitive behavioural therapies or family therapy. These psychological therapies focus specifically on maintaining abstinence and promoting behaviour change.

Alcohol withdrawal

Alcohol withdrawal typically occurs in dependent drinkers (>15 units per day) when alcohol consumption is stopped abruptly. Patients develop confusion, hallucinations, agitation, tremor and occasionally seizures. The extreme is delirium tremens. All patients at risk of withdrawal and wanting to stop drinking should undergo supervised detoxification. Although detoxification can be successfully undertaken in the community, in patients who have had previous seizures, have significant comorbidity, acute illness or lack of social support, hospital admission for withdrawal management is advocated.

Withdrawal is commonly managed with a reducing course of benzodiazepines (e.g. chlordiazepoxide or lorazepam) in accordance with local hospital protocols. In severe withdrawal, haloperidol or olanzapine may also be prescribed to control visual hallucinations. On the ward, patients are monitored for hallucinations, confusion, seizures and tremor and dosage adjusted accordingly. Withdrawal can be monitored formally using the Clinical Institute Withdrawal Assessment Scale (CIWA-Ar). After a successful withdrawal, in those with moderate to severe alcohol dependence, consider medical therapy with acamprosate, naltrexone or disulfiram to support abstinence in combination with counselling to prevent relapse.

Prevention of Wernicke–Korsakoff syndrome

High-dose thiamine should be offered to all hazardous drinkers to prevent the development of Wernicke–Korsakoff syndrome. Wernicke's encephalopathy is defined by as a classic triad of symptoms: mental confusion, ataxia and ophthalmoplegia. Korsakoff's psychosis is a late manifestation of the condition when Wernicke's encephalopathy has been treated inadequately. Those with malnutrition, decompensated chronic liver disease or acute alcohol withdrawal are at an increased risk of developing Wernicke–Korsakoff syndrome.

Management: A course of intravenous thiamine (Pabrinex®) is given followed by long-term oral prophylaxis.

27 Fatty liver disease

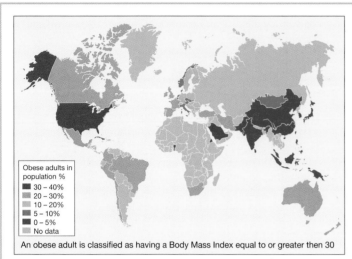

Obese adults in population %
30 – 40%
20 – 30%
10 – 20%
5 – 10%
0 – 5%
No data
An obese adult is classified as having a Body Mass Index equal to or greater then 30

Map 27-1 Global incidence of obesity.

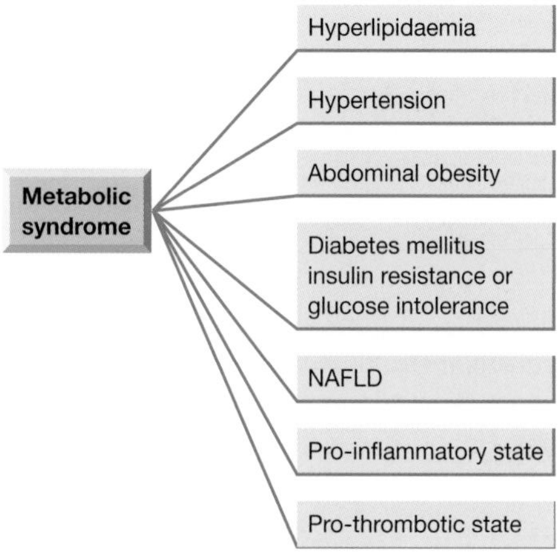

Metabolic syndrome
Hyperlipidaemia
Hypertension
Abdominal obesity
Diabetes mellitus insulin resistance or glucose intolerance
NAFLD
Pro-inflammatory state
Pro-thrombotic state

Figure 27-1 Features of metabolic syndrome.

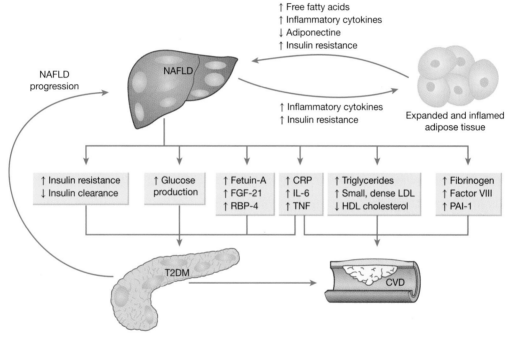

↑ Free fatty acids
↑ Inflammatory cytokines
↓ Adiponectine
↑ Insulin resistance
NAFLD progression
NAFLD
↑ Inflammatory cytokines
↑ Insulin resistance
Expanded and inflamed adipose tissue
↑ Insulin resistance
↓ Insulin clearance
↑ Glucose production
↑ Fetuin-A
↑ FGF-21
↑ RBP-4
↑ CRP
↑ IL-6
↑ TNF
↑ Triglycerides
↑ Small, dense LDL
↓ HDL cholesterol
↑ Fibrinogen
↑ Factor VIII
↑ PAI-1
T2DM
CVD

Figure 27-2 Mechanisms underlying the links between NAFLD, type II diabetes (T2DM) and cardiovascular disease (CVD).
NAFLD is common in those with T2DM, but may also precede the development of T2DM. T2DM is also a known risk factor for the progression of NAFLD to advanced liver disease and sometimes hepatocellular carcinoma (HCC).
Source: *Anstee QM et al. (2013) Reproduced with permission of Nature Publishing Group.*

Hepatology at a Glance, First Edition. Deepak Joshi, Geri Keane and Alison Brind.

Definitions

Non-alcoholic fatty liver disease (NAFLD): Encompasses a range of conditions from simple hepatic steatosis through to steatohepatitis and cirrhosis. The histological changes seen in NAFLD are identical to those in alcoholic liver disease; therefore NAFLD should only be diagnosed in those drinking less than 2 units of alcohol per day.

Non-alcoholic steatohepatitis (NASH): Presence of hepatic steatosis and inflammation with hepatocellular injury with or without fibrosis. NASH can progress to cirrhosis, liver failure and liver cancer.

NASH cirrhosis: Presence of cirrhosis with current or previous histological evidence of steatosis or steatohepatitis.

Epidemiology

In Europe, it is estimated 12–18% of the population have NAFLD, and of those 3–16% have NASH. The incidence of NAFLD is increasing and it is now the most common cause of liver disease in Western populations and an increasingly common indication for liver transplantation. Risk factors for NASH include obesity, diabetes, metabolic syndrome, male sex, old age and ethnicity.

Pathophysiology

NAFLD is increasingly recognised as the hepatic component of the multisystemic metabolic syndrome (Figures 27.1 and 27.2). In some cases, hepatic steatosis causes hepatocellular injury (ballooning of the hepatocytes and inflammatory infiltrate), leading to fibrosis, cirrhosis and ultimately HCC. However, why progression of the disease only occurs in a minority of patients with NAFLD remains unclear. A potential explanation is that progression occurs following a second liver injury ('second hit'), which is triggered by oxidative stress, mitochondrial abnormalities, TNF-α or changes in hormones, such as adiponectin and leptin. Ultimately, this results in the activation of hepatic stellate cells, which produce collagen, leading to fibrosis and cirrhosis.

Investigations
Blood tests

The majority of patients with NAFLD are asymptomatic and are identified incidentally because of abnormal liver biochemistry (typically a raised GGT or ALT). In NAFLD, liver biochemistry may be normal. As the disease progresses ALT levels often fall and AST levels rise, the AST : ALT ratio can be useful in guiding disease severity. Jaundice is rare and typically only a feature of end-stage liver disease in the presence of NASH cirrhosis. Up to 60% have an elevated serum ferritin, which reflects an acute phase response due to hepatic injury rather than iron overload.

Ultrasound

Up to one-third of the population in the UK have evidence of hepatic steatosis on ultrasound. Although an ultrasound scan can identify the radiological features of advanced fibrosis or cirrhosis it cannot reliably differentiate simple fatty liver disease from NASH.

Biopsy

A liver biopsy is the only definitive way of excluding NASH. However, it is impractical to perform a liver biopsy on everyone with NAFLD. Indications for a liver biopsy in NAFLD include unclear aetiology or uncertainty of the stage of liver disease. Currently, there are no non-invasive markers that can reliably identify steatohepatitis but clinical scores (e.g. the NAFLD Fibrosis Score), transient elastography and serum fibrosis markers are becoming increasingly accurate at staging fibrosis.

Management

Patients with NAFLD should be stratified into those with NASH/advanced fibrosis and those with steatosis alone. Patients with steatosis should be given lifestyle advice and discharged. Patients with NASH need multidisciplinary input to support implementation of lifestyle changes and medical treatment. Patients with advanced fibrosis require surveillance for hepatocellular carcinoma, oesophageal varices and features of decompensation.

Lifestyle management and weight loss

All patients with fatty liver disease without decompensation should be strongly recommended to modify their diet by reducing sugar and fat intake and increasing exercise levels so they gradually lose weight (aim >10% loss of body mass). Dietetic support is often useful.

Medical management

Most patients with NAFLD have additional systemic complications of obesity and metabolic syndrome. Therefore they should be screened and treated for cardiovascular risk factors (e.g. hypertension or hyperlipidaemia). Statin-induced hepatoxicity has not been shown to be more common in NAFLD. These drugs can therefore be prescribed safely if required and may have additional beneficial effects on the liver.

Other therapies such as metformin, peroxisome proliferator-activated receptors γ (PPAR-γ) agonists (pioglitazone and rosiglitazone), glucagon like peptide-1 analogues (exenatide) and dipeptidyl peptidase-4 inhibitors (sitagliptan) have been shown to be effective in improving liver biochemistry but not fibrosis. Metformin also reduces HCC risk. Long-term high dose vitamin E (800 IU/day) may improve certain histological features of NASH but again will not improve established fibrosis. However, cautious use is advised, as it has been associated with haemorrhagic stroke and prostate cancer.

Surgical management

Bariatric surgery has been proven to be highly effective treatment for patients with NASH, resulting in a reduction in steatohepatitis and liver fibrosis in nearly all patients. A concurrent reduction in weight and diabetic medication requirements is also seen. Bariatric surgical options include gastric balloons, gastric banding and bypass surgery (see Chapter 42). These treatments are cost-effective and should be considered in those who are morbidly obese.

Prognosis

Patients with NAFLD have a good prognosis. However, those with NASH have a 5–20% risk of progression to cirrhosis within 10 years. Overall mortality results from complications of advanced liver disease and cardiovascular manifestations of the underlying metabolic syndrome. Obesity and NAFLD are strongly associated with HCC; prevalence is estimated to be <0.5% in NAFLD and 2.8% in NASH.

28 Hepatitis A and hepatitis E viruses

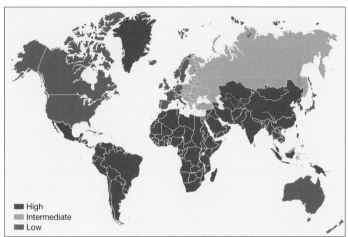

Map 28-1 Global distribution of chronic hepatitis A virus infection.

High
Intermediate
Low

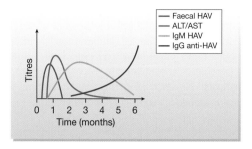

Figure 28-1 Acute hepatitis A serology.

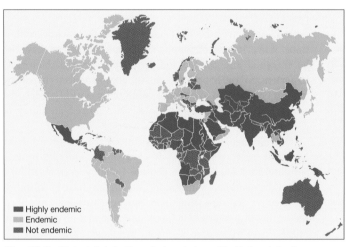

Map 28-2 Global distribution of chronic hepatitis E virus infection.

Highly endemic
Endemic
Not endemic

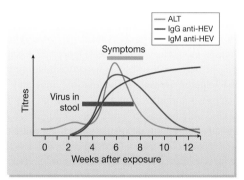

Figure 28-2 Acute hepatitis E serology.

Hepatology at a Glance, First Edition. Deepak Joshi, Geri Keane and Alison Brind.
© 2015 John Wiley & Sons, Ltd. Published 2015 by John Wiley & Sons, Ltd. Companion website: www.ataglanceseries.com/hepatology

Hepatitis A virus

Hepatitis A virus (HAV) is a RNA virus. Transmission is through direct person–person contact, contaminated water, shellfish taken from contaminated water or contaminated foods. HAV is shed in the faeces of infected people. HAV is more prevalent in lower socio-economic groups due to poor sanitation and hygiene. HAV infection is common in the developing world and less common in developed countries, although outbreaks have been described.

Risk factors for HAV infection

- Travel to a high risk area (see Map 28.1) (50% of cases);
- Sexual or household contact with HAV infected person (10%);
- Men who have sex with men (9%);
- Food or infected water outbreak (8%).

Diagnosis

The incubation period is 2–6 weeks (mean 28 days) with jaundice, nausea, fever, fatigue and lethargy, although patients may be asymptomatic. Diagnosis is made by detecting serum IgM anti-HAV. HAV is present in the stool at the incubation period. Infection does not result in chronic infection or chronic liver disease. Acute liver failure is rare. Treatment is usually supportive.

Vaccination

Incidence of HAV has declined since the introduction of vaccines. Two types of vaccines are available: a live attenuated vaccine and an inactivated vaccine. After the first dose, protection is evident 2–4 weeks later. After the second booster injection immunity is provided for more than 20 years.

Hepatitis E virus

Hepatitis E virus (HEV) is an RNA virus that accounts for more than 3 million cases of acute hepatitis worldwide, resulting in over 70 000 deaths. Rarely, HEV can also lead to a chronic hepatitis. Four genotypes have been identified in humans: genotype 1, Asia, Africa and South America; genotype 2, Central America and Africa; genotype 4, Japan and China. HEV genotypes 3 and 4 infect both humans and pigs and are highly prevalent in developed countries with large pig populations.

Transmission

Most transmission is via the faecal–oral route especially with HEV genotypes 1 and 2. HEV genotype 3 infection is zoonotic (transmission from animals to humans). Transmission is also possible through contaminated blood products.

Clinical presentation

Middle-aged men are more often affected. The vast majority of patients with HEV infection remain asymptomatic. Typical manifestations include jaundice, fever, malaise, myalgia, vomiting and abdominal pain; rarely, acute liver failure. Extrahepatic manifestations, in particular neurological manifestations, are well described. These include presentation with Guillain–Barre, encephalitis, polyradiculopathy, brachial neuritis and myopathy. Chronic HEV infection has also been associated with the development of glomerulonephritis and cryoglobulinaemia.

Diagnosis

Incubation period ranges 2–9 weeks. Diagnosis is based on the detection of anti-HEV IgM. HEV RNA is detectable in both blood and stool; the virus can be detected in the stool for up to 2 weeks. Liver biochemistry demonstrates an acute hepatitis (increased AST/ALT).

Special patient populations

Pregnancy

Pregnant women are more susceptible to HEV infection. HEV infection is the most common viral cause of acute liver failure in pregnancy. Poorer maternal and fetal outcomes are described in pregnant women who develop HEV infection and jaundice. Infection is common in the second or third trimester (median gestational age 28 weeks).

Chronic liver disease

HEV can result in a chronic hepatitis. Cirrhosis caused by HEV has not been described. HEV 'superinfection' can occur in patients with chronic liver disease, resulting in hepatic decompensation.

Immunosuppressed patients

Chronic HEV infection has been reported in kidney, liver and heart transplant recipients and HIV patients with CD4 counts <200 cells/mm. A HEV RNA should be performed in any such patient with a persistent transaminitis.

Treatment

Acute HEV infection in immunocompetent patients is self-limiting and care is usually supportive.

In immunosuppressed patients, attempts should be made to reduce immunosuppression. Overall, limited data are available in the treatment of HEV with antiviral therapy but ribavirin (600–1000 mg/day) for 3 months may be given if reduction in immunosuppression fails.

Vaccination

Remains in development phase although one vaccine has been recently licensed in China.

Other viruses

Cytomegalovirus (CMV) infection can cause an acute hepatitis, more common and frequent in immunocompromised patients. Agents such as ganciclovir, valganciclovir and foscarnet can be used. Herpes simplex virus (HSV) types 1 and 2 infection can cause a hepatitis and more rarely acute liver failure. Patients at risk include neonates, immunosuppressed patients and pregnant women. Oral and genital lesions may only be present in 30% of patients. Treatment is with aciclovir.

29 Hepatitis B virus and delta hepatitis

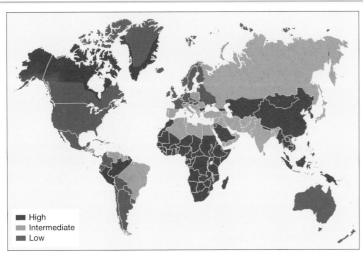

Figure 29-1 Global distribution of chronic hepatitis B virus infection.

High
Intermediate
Low

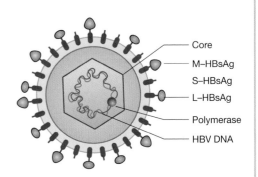

Figure 29-2 HBV structure.

Core
M–HBsAg
S–HBsAg
L–HBsAg
Polymerase
HBV DNA

Figure 29-3 Natural history of HBV infection.

Disease status: Immunotolerant | Active | Non-replicative | Reactivation

HBV DNA: HBsAg + | HBsAg –

Exposure

ALT: HBeAg + | Anti-HBe+

Exposure

Time

Table 29-1 Interpretation of HBV serology.

HBsAg	HBsAb	HBcAb (total)	HBcAb IgM	HBeAg	HBeAb	Interpretation
–	–	–	–			No previous infection Vaccination required
+		+	+			Possible acute HBV
+	–	+	+/–	+	+/–	Chronic HBV eAg +ve disease
+	–	+	+/–	–	+/–	Chronic HBV eAg –ve disease
–	+/–	+				Previous HBV exposure with recovery or immunity
–	–	+				Previous HBV exposure or immunity

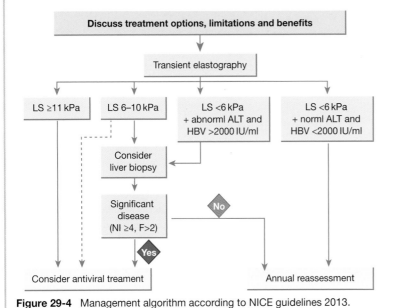

Figure 29-4 Management algorithm according to NICE guidelines 2013.

Discuss treatment options, limitations and benefits

Transient elastography

LS ≥11 kPa | LS 6–10 kPa | LS <6 kPa + abnorml ALT and HBV >2000 IU/ml | LS <6 kPa + norml ALT and HBV <2000 IU/ml

Consider liver biopsy

Significant disease (NI ≥4, F>2) — No

Yes

Consider antiviral treatment

Annual reassessment

Box 29-1 Thresholds for treatment

- Adults >30 years with HBV DNA >2000 IU/ml and abnormal ALT 3 months apart
- HBV DNA >20 000 IU/ml and abnormal ALT 3 months apart
- All patients with cirrhosis and detectable HBV DNA regardless of HBV DNA and ALT levels

Hepatology at a Glance, First Edition. Deepak Joshi, Geri Keane and Alison Brind.
© 2015 John Wiley & Sons, Ltd. Published 2015 by John Wiley & Sons, Ltd. Companion website: www.ataglanceseries.com/hepatology

Hepatitis B virus
Epidemiology

Over 350 million people are infected worldwide with chronic hepatitis B virus infection (CHBV). Endemic areas include sub-Saharan Africa and South-East Asia (15% prevalence). Most global infection is transmitted vertically, from infected mothers during delivery, or acquired in early childhood. It is not transmitted by breastfeeding. Sexual transmission and intravenous drug use are more common in Western countries. CHBV is one of the leading causes of cirrhosis and hepatocellular carcinoma. Eight genotypes (A–H) have been identified with distinct geographical correlation: A, Northern Europe, North America, Central Africa; B, South-East Asia and Japan; C, South-East Asia; D, Southern Europe, India E, West Africa; F, South/Central America.

Structure

The HBV virion or Dane particle is 42 nm and consists of a nucleocapsid (core) surrounded by an outer envelope of surface protein (HBsAg). The protein core (HBcAg) contains an incomplete double-stranded circular DNA and DNA polymerase/reverse transcriptase. HBV DNA contains genes that encode structural (surface (s), core (c) and replicative proteins (polymerase and X)). HBeAg is a protein that is formed from self-cleavage of the pre-core–core gene product. HBV is not a cytopathic virus and mediates liver injury through cytotoxic T-lymphocyte-mediated lysis of infected hepatocytes. HBV-DNA persists in the nucleus as cccDNA.

Mutations

HBeAg negative infection arises due to mutations. Mutations can also arise in the DNA polymerase, especially in patients on antiviral therapy.

Clinical features and natural history
Acute HBV

Most patients are asymptomatic but many develop jaundice, fever or lethargy. ALF is rare. Some 95% of adults will clear the virus and develop immunitybut 5% of adults will develop CHBV infection.

Chronic HBV

CHBV (HBsAg positive >6 months) is usually asymptomatic. There are several types of CHBV infection:
• *Immune tolerant*: HBeAg positive, high HBV DNA, normal aminotransferases, mild necro-inflammation on liver biopsy. Highly contagious. Usually occurs with infection acquired in childhood. Potential to seroconvert spontaneously (loss of HBeAg and HBsAg).
• *Immune reactive*: HBeAg positive, lower HBV DNA, fluctuating aminotransferases, moderate necro-inflammation on liver biopsy, higher risk of fibrosis Usually occurs when infected in adulthood.
• *HBeAg negative CHBV*: HBeAg negative, anti-HBeAb positive, fluctuating HBV DNA >1000 IU/mL, fluctuating aminotransferases. High risk of progressive fibrosis and cirrhosis, complications of chronic liver disease and HCC.
• *Reactivation*: precipitated by immunosuppression and/or chemotherapy. HBsAg negative, HBcAb positive, fluctuating HBV DNA, fluctuating aminotransferases.
• *Occult HBV infection*: HBsAg negative, low HBV DNA (<200 IU/mL). Clinical relevance remains unclear.

Investigations

A full history and examination is required. Special consideration should be given to ethnic origin, a family history of cirrhosis or HCC and previous HBV therapy. Extrahepatic manifestations occur in 1 in 10 patients and include membranous glomerulonephritis, vasculitis, polyarteritis nodosa, cryoglobulinaemia and aplastic anaemia.
• Liver function tests: consider acute HBV or reactivation if AST/ALT >1000 IU/mL;
• HBV serology (see Table 29.1);
• HBV DNA by polymerase chain reaction;
• HAV, HCV, HDV and HIV serology given similar transmission routes;
• Liver US scan;
• Consider Fibroscan or liver biopsy.

Management
Vaccination

Should be offered to the following patient groups: health care professionals, men who have sex with men (MSM), sexual partners or close family living with an infected person, travellers to high-risk areas, patients with kidney disease or receiving haemodialysis. Babies born to mothers who are HBeAg positive should receive both active (HBsAg) and passive vaccination (hepatitis B immunoglobulin) after delivery. Babies born to HBeAg negative mothers should receive active vaccination.

General

• *Acute HBV*: for cases of ALF consider oral antiviral therapy.
• *CHBV*: goal is to suppress HBV DNA, induce HBeAg clearance, HBsAg clearance and prevent HCC and cirrhosis.

Antivirals

Immunomodulatory agents (e.g. pegylated interferon): Recommended for HBeAg positive patients, age <60 years, HBV DNA <10^8 IU/mL, genotype A or B, non-cirrhotic, ALT >3× ULN. Treatment is for 48 weeks.

Oral antiviral therapy (e.g. entecavir and tenofovir): Lamivudine monotherapy is no longer recommended as first-line therapy due to the development of resistance. Tenofovir and entecavir are both highly potent antivirals with high barriers to resistance. Tenofovir requires renal monitoring. Entecavir is not recommended for patients with previous lamivudine resistance. Treatment is often lifelong but may be withdrawn after loss of HBsAg or in HBeAb after prolonged HBV-DNA negativity.

Special considerations

• *Cirrhosis secondary to HBV*: treat long-term with oral antiviral therapies irrespective of eAg status and HBV DNA level (unless negative).
• *HBV in pregnancy*: mothers with HBV DNA viral load >10^6 IU/mL require treatment after 28 weeks' gestation with oral antiviral therapy.
• *Patients undergoing chemotherapy/antibody induction*: HBV reactivation can occur worse with haematological chemotherapy. Prophylaxis is recommended in HBsAg positive patients with oral antivirals at least 6 months after chemotherapy. HBcAb should have active monitoring.
• *HIV–HBV co-infection*: patients should not be treated with single agents. Include antiviral therapy that treats both infections (e.g. tenofovir).
• Surveillance for HCC with 6-monthly US scans and AFP for patients with cirrhosis or strong family history of HCC.

Delta hepatitis virus

HDV is an RNA virus that requires HBV in order to replicate. Approximately 5% of HBV carriers are co-infected with HDV. HDV can occur as a superinfection in a patient with HBV or as a chronic infection leading to a more aggressive course.

Investigations

All patients with HBV should be screened with anti-HDV. Anti-HDV IgM (acute infection), anti-HDV IgG (chronic infection), HDV RNA PCR. HBV viral loads are lower in cases of HBV–HDV co-infection compared to HBV mono-infection.

Management

Antiviral therapy with PEG-IFN for 48 weeks has been shown to reduce viral load. Patients require surveillance for HCC. Patients with cirrhosis secondary to HDV–HBV are eligible for liver transplantation.

30 Hepatitis C virus

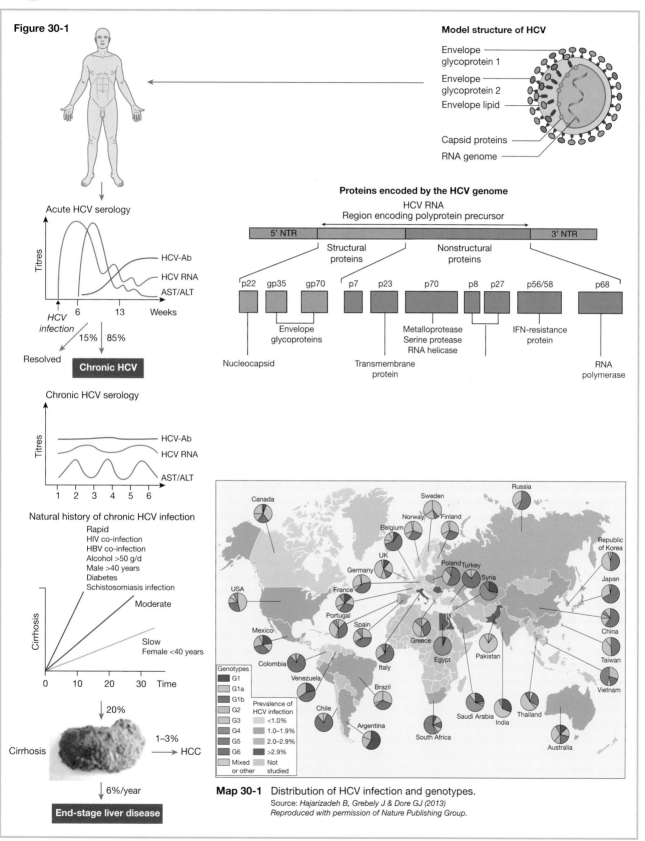

Figure 30-1

Model structure of HCV

Envelope glycoprotein 1
Envelope glycoprotein 2
Envelope lipid
Capsid proteins
RNA genome

Acute HCV serology

Titres

HCV-Ab
HCV RNA
AST/ALT

6   13   Weeks

HCV infection

Resolved   15%   85%

Chronic HCV

Chronic HCV serology

Titres

HCV-Ab
HCV RNA
AST/ALT

1 2 3 4 5 6

Proteins encoded by the HCV genome

HCV RNA
Region encoding polyprotein precursor

5' NTR   Structural proteins   Nonstructural proteins   3' NTR

p22 gp35 gp70   p7 p23   p70   p8 p27   p56/58   p68

Envelope glycoproteins

Metalloprotease
Serine protease
RNA helicase

IFN-resistance protein

Nucleocapsid

Transmembrane protein

RNA polymerase

Natural history of chronic HCV infection

Rapid
HIV co-infection
HBV co-infection
Alcohol >50 g/d
Male >40 years
Diabetes
Schistosomiasis infection

Cirrhosis

Moderate

Slow
Female <40 years

0   10   20   30   Time

↓ 20%

Cirrhosis   1–3% → HCC

↓ 6%/year

End-stage liver disease

Map 30-1 Distribution of HCV infection and genotypes.
Source: Hajarizadeh B, Grebely J & Dore GJ (2013)
Reproduced with permission of Nature Publishing Group.

Genotypes
G1
G1a
G1b
G2
G3
G4
G5
G6
Mixed or other

Prevalence of HCV infection
<1.0%
1.0–1.9%
2.0–2.9%
>2.9%
Not studied

Hepatology at a Glance, First Edition. Deepak Joshi, Geri Keane and Alison Brind.
© 2015 John Wiley & Sons, Ltd. Published 2015 by John Wiley & Sons, Ltd. Companion website: www.ataglanceseries.com/hepatology

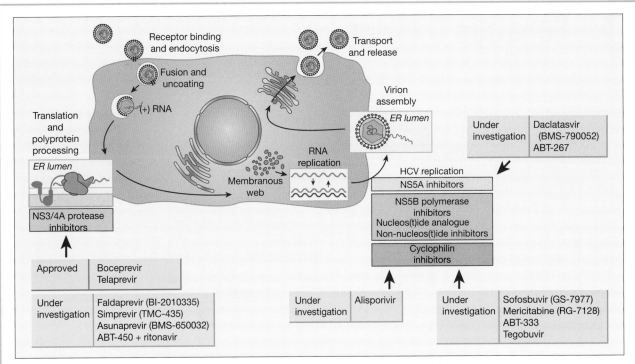

Figure 30-2 HCV replication and mechanism of action of new directly acting anti-virals (DAAs).

Table 30-1

Drug	Common side effects	Management
Pegylated interferon	Flu-like symptoms WCC Haemoglobin Depression Fatigue	Usually improves 6–8 weeks after starting Reduce dose ± GCSF Reduce dose ± EPO ± blood transfusion Addition of SSRI
Ribavirin	Haemoglobin (secondary to haemolysis)	Reduce dose ± EPO ± blood transfusion
Telaprevir	Haemoglobin Rash Pruritis	EPO ± blood transfusion
Boceprevir	Haemoglobin Metallic taste (dysgeusia)	EPO ± blood transfusion

Hepatitis C virus

Hepatitis C virus (HCV) was first characterised in 1988.

Epidemiology

A total of 3–4 million people are infected every year. The global prevalence of chronic HCV is estimated to be 130–170 million people. Countries with high prevalence rates of chronic infection include Egypt (22%), Pakistan (5%) and China (3%). In developed countries the prevalence rate (HCV Ab positive) is estimated to be less than 2%. Transmission is via contaminated blood post-transfusion, contaminated needles in intravenous drug use and medical therapy. Vertical transmission is low. No vaccines are available for prevention of HCV. High-risk groups include blood recipients of non-screened blood, intravenous drug users (IVDUs), persons from areas of high prevalence, individuals with high-risk sexual behaviours, incarcerated

persons, men who have sex with men (MSM), patients co-infected with HIV.

Structure and replication

HCV is a small enveloped RNA virus. It has six genotypes (1–6) with further subtypes (a,b,c). The genome consists of an open reading frame that lacks a proof-reading function for the RNA-dependent RNA polymerase. This accounts for the high mutation rate and genetic variability (quasispecies). Replication occurs within hepatocytes. HCV can infect dendritic cells, lymphocytes, monocytes and B cells.

Pathogenesis

HCV can cause direct liver injury or indirect liver injury through immune-mediated pathways. Pathways related to necrosis, apoptosis, angiogenesis are all up-regulated leading to progressive fibrosis.

Clinical features and natural history

Acute HCV

Usually asymptomatic or non-specific symptoms (e.g. lethargy, malaise, pyrexia). HCV RNA is detectable within 1–2 weeks before viral titres peak at 8 weeks. Jaundice at the time of acute infection is associated with a decreased risk of chronic infection. HCV antibody (Ab) is detectable within 20–150 days post-exposure. Some 85% will develop chronic infection.

Chronic HCV

HCV Ab positive and detectable HCV RNA for at least 6 months after acute infection. Those with co-infection with HIV and IVDUs are at higher risk of chronic infection.

Most patients remain asymptomatic although chronic infection is usually asymptomatic but can be associated with fatigue. Chronic HCV infection is characterised by progressive fibrosis with the development of cirrhosis (30% over 10–20 years, 30% over 20–30 years and in 30% over 30 years), liver failure and HCC. HCV-related cirrhosis is complicated by decompensation 1% per annum and a leading cause of HCC, a rate of 1–3% per annum. Factors associated with rapid fibrosis progression include: male gender, older age at time of infection, alcohol excess, metabolic syndrome with hepatic steatosis/diabetes, HIV or HBV co-infection, shistosomiasis infection co-infection.

Extrahepatic manifestations

Direct infection of B cells is thought to be responsible for the associated B-cell-related lymphomas and cryoglobulinaemia. Cryoglobulinaemia is a vasculitis affecting the small and medium-sized vessels and can present with purpura and glomerulonephritis peripheral ulceration. The presence of cryoglobulins in a patient with chronic HCV is an indication for antiviral therapy. Can be associated with Sjögren's syndrome and diabetes mellitus.

Investigations

General

- HCV Ab, HCV RNA, HCV genotype, HBV, HIV serology;
- Liver biopsy, Fibroscan or fibrosis markers to assess degree of fibrosis.

Additional

- *Interleukin-28B (IL-28B):* polymorphisms in this gene are associated with spontaneous clearance of acute HCV and sustained virologic response (SVR) in with treatment with pegylated interferon (PEG-IFN) and ribavirin in patients with genotype 1.
- *Cryoglobulins:* blood sample needs to be stored on ice and taken to the laboratory immediately.

Treatment

All patients should be considered for antiviral therapy. Other co-morbidities (e.g. diabetes mellitus and hypertension) should be optimised pre-treatment and patients advised to abstain from alcohol. The goal of treatment is an SVR negative HCV RNA 24 week post-therapy (although SVR 12 weeks is now being considered indicative of cure).

Acute HCV

- Important to treat early as SVR >80%.
- Check HCV RNA every 4 weeks. Patients remaining viraemic should be treated within 3 months.
- Treatment is with subcutaneous PEG-IFN 180 µg/week and oral ribavirin for 24–48 weeks irrespective of viral genotype.

Chronic HCV

- *Genotype 1:* PEG-IFN/ribavirin + protease inhibitor (boceprevir or telaprevir) for 24–48 weeks.
- *Non-genotype 1:* PEG-IFN/ribavirin for 24–48 weeks remains the standard of care.

The treatment of chronic HCV is changing rapidly with new oral directly acting antivirals (DAAs) being rapidly developed. DAAs target different viral proteins (see Figure 30.2). DAAs are being used both with and without PEG-IFN and ribavirin. Some are genotype-specific (e.g. telaprevir and boceprevir) and some are pan-genotypic (e.g. sofusbuvir). SVR rates are anticipated to be greater than 90%.

Factors predictive of an SVR with PEG-IFN and ribavirin:

- *Pre-treatment:* non-genotype 1, low baseline HCV viral load, IL-28B genotype (CC > CT > TT), White race, minimal fibrosis, age <40 years, female sex;
- *On treatment:* rapid virological response > early virological response, adherence to treatment, achieving maximal doses of treatment.

Autoimmune hepatitis

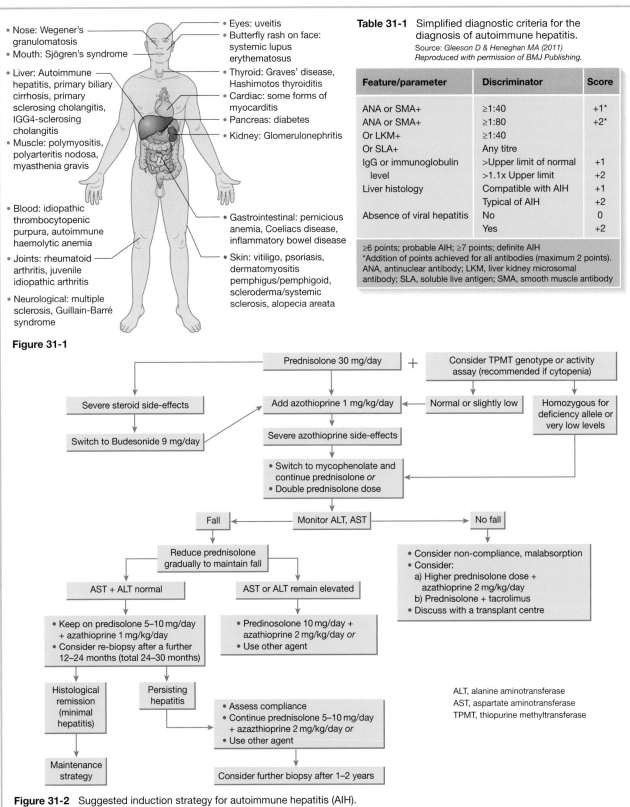

- Nose: Wegener's granulomatosis
- Mouth: Sjögren's syndrome
- Liver: Autoimmune hepatitis, primary biliary cirrhosis, primary sclerosing cholangitis, IGG4-sclerosing cholangitis
- Muscle: polymyositis, polyarteritis nodosa, myasthenia gravis

- Blood: idiopathic thrombocytopenic purpura, autoimmune haemolytic anemia
- Joints: rheumatoid arthritis, juvenile idiopathic arthritis
- Neurological: multiple sclerosis, Guillain-Barré syndrome

- Eyes: uveitis
- Butterfly rash on face: systemic lupus erythematosus
- Thyroid: Graves' disease, Hashimotos thyroiditis
- Cardiac: some forms of myocarditis
- Pancreas: diabetes
- Kidney: Glomerulonephritis

- Gastrointestinal: pernicious anemia, Coeliacs disease, inflammatory bowel disease
- Skin: vitiligo, psoriasis, dermatomyositis pemphigus/pemphigoid, scleroderma/systemic sclerosis, alopecia areata

Figure 31-1

Table 31-1 Simplified diagnostic criteria for the diagnosis of autoimmune hepatitis.

Source: Gleeson D & Heneghan MA (2011)
Reproduced with permission of BMJ Publishing.

Feature/parameter	Discriminator	Score
ANA or SMA+	≥1:40	+1*
ANA or SMA+	≥1:80	+2*
Or LKM+	≥1:40	
Or SLA+	Any titre	
IgG or immunoglobulin level	>Upper limit of normal	+1
	>1.1x Upper limit	+2
Liver histology	Compatible with AIH	+1
	Typical of AIH	+2
Absence of viral hepatitis	No	0
	Yes	+2

≥6 points; probable AIH; ≥7 points; definite AIH
*Addition of points achieved for all antibodies (maximum 2 points).
ANA, antinuclear antibody; LKM, liver kidney microsomal antibody; SLA, soluble live antigen; SMA, smooth muscle antibody

ALT, alanine aminotransferase
AST, aspartate aminotransferase
TPMT, thiopurine methyltransferase

Figure 31-2 Suggested induction strategy for autoimmune hepatitis (AIH).

Source: Gleeson D & Heneghan MA (2011)
Reproduced with permission of BMJ Publishing.

Hepatology at a Glance, First Edition. Deepak Joshi, Geri Keane and Alison Brind.
© 2015 John Wiley & Sons, Ltd. Published 2015 by John Wiley & Sons, Ltd. Companion website: www.ataglanceseries.com/hepatology

Autoimmune hepatitis

Autoimmune hepatitis (AIH) is a chronic, progressive, inflammatory disease that without treatment results in end-stage liver disease.

Epidemiology

AIH is the second most common autoimmune hepatopathy after PBC. Incidence is 10–17 per 100 000 population. More than 80% of patients are female and up to half have another autoimmune condition (e.g. Hashimoto's thyroiditis, inflammatory bowel disease or diabetes; see Figure 31.1).

Pathogenesis

The immunopathogenesis of AIH is unknown, but onset maybe triggered by drugs (e.g. nitrofuratoin or minocycline) or a virus (e.g. hepatitis A, CMV) in a genetically susceptible individual.

Clinical presentation

Common presenting features include fatigue, nausea, weight loss, jaundice and, rarely, fulminant liver failure. Some 25% of patients are asymptomatic.

Diagnostic criteria

AIH has no pathognomonic features and diagnosis is dependent on a combination of biochemical, immunological and pathological features in the absence of other liver disease. Blood tests typically demonstrate an elevated ALT and AST, raised serum immunoglobulins, negative viral serology and raised autoantibodies (antinuclear antibody, ANA, and anti-smooth muscle antibody, ASMA). IgG is elevated in 85%. IgA is rarely elevated in AIH and if raised is more suggestive of ALD, NAFLD or drug-induced liver injury. Alkaline phosphatase is often normal and if elevated is suggestive of an overlap syndrome (see Chapter 34). If only some features of AIH are present, full and simplified diagnostic criteria, developed by the International Autoimmune Hepatitis Group (IAIHG) can be used to aid diagnosis (see Table 31.1). A score of >7 is 80% sensitive and 97% specific for AIH.

A liver biopsy is recommended in all patients with suspected AIH unless there is significant comorbidity or contraindication. Some 20% of patients identified as having AIH based on scoring and clinical criteria alone, will ultimately be found to have NAFLD. Histological features of AIH include portal mononuclear cell infiltration and interface hepatitis (also present in drug-induced, viral and other hepatitides). In addition, up to one-third will have evidence of cirrhosis at the time of diagnosis.

Trial of steroids: When the diagnosis continues to remain equivocal despite clinical investigations and IAIHG scoring, a trial of corticosteroids can be considered. If the transaminases do not fall AIH is much less likely.

Categories

AIH can be divided in to two distinct subtypes: types 1 and 2. Type 1 is associated with the presence of ANA and smooth muscle antibody (SMA) whereas type 2 is characterised by the presence of either anti-liver kidney microsomal-1 (LKM-1) or anti-liver cytosolic-1 (LC-1) antibodies. Type 2 accounts for only 10% of cases in northern Europe and North America but is more common in Southern Europe. Type 2 tends to affect young adults and have a worse prognosis, with frequent relapses and greater numbers progressing to cirrhosis.

Management

Initial management: Immunosuppressive regimens for the initial treatment and maintenance of AIH are much debated. Current British Society of Gastroenterology (BSG) guidelines recommend initial treatment with 30 mg/day prednisolone tapering to 10 mg/day gradually over 2–3 months (as the transaminases fall) and commencing azathioprine (1–2 mg/kg/day), usually a few weeks after diagnosis and once the thiopurine methlytransferase (TPMT) result has been obtained to exclude TPMT homozygosity.

The ultimate treatment goal in AIH is to achieve complete normalisation of the transaminases, IgG and reduction of hepatic inflammation. If the ALT and AST do not fall, this is a prognostically poor sign. In this group, after 2 years of unsuccessful standard therapy, higher doses of immunosuppression can be considered. Sequential liver biopsies are often used to monitor response. Histological remission lags significantly behind biochemical remission in AIH, therefore continuation of a dosage of 5–10 mg/day prednisolone for 2 years and at least 12 months after normalisation of transaminases is advisable, if tolerated.

Relapse: Within 12 months of stopping treatment after biochemical and histological remission has been achieved 50–90% will relapse, signified by a peak in transaminases or a raised IAIHG score. Relapse is more common in certain groups (e.g. type 2 AIH). Routine maintenance therapy with azathioprine (1–2 mg/kg/day) is therefore recommended in all type 2 patients and in type 1 patients who relapse. In younger patients without relapse, maintenance immunosuppression therapy is also often continued to try and prevent progression to cirrhosis. Patients who relapse off treatment should be treated *de novo* and maintenance therapy with prednisolone and azathioprine continued long term.

Therapeutic side effects: Up to half of patients develop significant steroid side effects (e.g. cushingoid features, osteoporosis or diabetes). In these cases prednisolone can be swapped to budesonide (except in those with cirrhosis). Calcium and vitamin D supplements are recommended in all patients and a dual-energy X-ray absorptiometry (DEXA) scan should be performed every 1–5 years depending on risk factors. Azathioprine is rarely associated with bone marrow suppression and regular monitoring is advised while on treatment (weekly for 6 weeks, monthly for 6 months and 3-monthly thereafter).

HCC surveillance: 6-monthly AFP + US is advocated in cirrhotic patients with AIH. One-quarter of patients will have a raised AFP at diagnosis; this reflects acute liver inflammation and is rarely associated with HCC.

Prognosis

Approximately 10–20% of patients with AIH will ultimately require liver transplantation. Referral for transplant assessment should be considered in those with severe disease characterised by non-responsive transaminases, signs of decompensation or fulminant hepatic failure. AIH recurs in 20% of grafts post-transplantation. Five-year survival following transplantation is approximately 75%.

32 Primary biliary cirrhosis

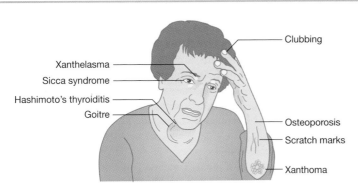

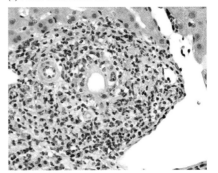

(a) Focal duct obliteration

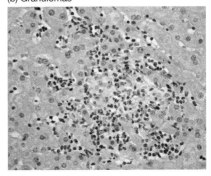

(b) Granulomas

Table 32-1

PBC stage	Histological features
Stage 1	Inflammation or connective tissue abnormality of the portal areas
Stage 2	Fibrosis and/or inflammation of the portal or periportal areas
Stage 3	Bridging fibrosis
Stage 4	Cirrhosis

Table 32-2   Mayo risk prediction model (predicts survival in PBC over next 7 years)

Mayo Score = 0.04 (age) + 0.87 log (bilirubin) − 2.53 log (albumin) + 2.38 log (prothrombin time) +0.86 (oedema score)

Oedema score:
0 = no oedema without diuretics
1 = oedema with diuretics
0.5 = otherwise

Web page for online calculator:
http://www.mayoclinic.org/medical-professionals/model-end-stage-liver-disease/natural-history-model-for-primary-biliary-cirrhosis

Primary biliary cirrhosis

Primary biliary cirrhosis (PBC) is an autoimmune disease of the small intrahepatic bile ducts.

Epidemiology

PBC is the most common autoimmune hepatopathy with a prevalence of 25–40 per 100 000 population. More than 90% of patients are female and onset is typically in middle age. It is associated with other autoimmune disorders (e.g. Sjögren's syndrome/Sicca syndrome, Hashimoto's thyroiditis, CREST/Raynaud's phenomenon and coeliac disease).

Pathogenesis

Aetiology is unknown but is thought to arise as a result of genetic predisposition combined with environmental triggers.

Clinical presentation

Patients can present with pruritus, lethargy or decompensation. However, many are diagnosed as a result of asymptomatic abnormal liver biochemistry. Clinical signs include xanthalasma, hepatomegaly, clubbing and excoriations due to pruritus.

Investigations

PBC is characterised by cholestatic LFTs, positive anti-mitochondrial antibodies (AMA) and a raised IgM. AMA against the M2 antigen (the enzyme PDC-E2) which is specific for PBC and present in 95% of patients and <1% of the unaffected population. In AMA negative cases, ANA is highly specific marker (>95%). ANA is directed against the nuclear body or envelope proteins such as anti-Sp100 and anti-gp210, which are present as multiple nuclear dots and peri-nuclear rims, respectively. Anti-smooth muscle antibody (ASMA) is also often present.

A liver biopsy is no longer regarded as necessary to diagnose PBC but may be required in those without classic serology. Histological features include a non-suppurative cholangitis and focal duct obliteration with granuloma formation (termed the florid duct lesion), which is pathognomonic of PBC. There are four histological stages of PBC, which are based on the degree of bile duct damage, inflammation and fibrosis. Since the liver is not uniformly affected in PBC all four stages may be present in each biopsy; the most advanced feature determines stage.

A rise in bilirubin and fall in albumin and platelets are recognised as early indicators of the development of cirrhosis and portal hypertension.

Management

Ursodeoxycholic acid (UDCA): 10–15 mg/kg/day has a limited effect on symptoms (fatigue and lethargy) but improves liver biochemistry and pathology in early disease; histological progression to cirrhosis was significantly lower (7% vs 34%) in those receiving UCDA compared to no treatment. If ALP falls by >40% or normalises at 1 year ('Barcelona criteria') it is associated with a 95% transplant-free survival at 14 years. UCDA has no clear effect on survival or progression to transplantation in advanced disease.

Steroids and immunosuppressants: In PBC, like other autoimmune liver disease, steroids have been shown to improve liver biochemistry. However, due to their adverse effect on bone mineral density in long-term use, they are not routinely used. Other immunosuppressive agents like azathioprine, ciclosporin, methotrexate, chlorambucil and mycophenolate mofetil have been marginally effective but are reserved for refractory cases.

Fatigue: In PBC fatigue is recognised as a difficult symptom to manage and has a major impact on quality of life. It does not correlate with disease severity. It is strongly associated with autonomic dysfunction (in particular orthostatic hypotension and sleep disturbance, especially daytime somnolence). Measures to reduce these factors (e.g. reducing caffeine intake) have had some impact. Psychological support and antidepressants (e.g. fluoxetine) have also been used with some success. Hypothyroidism and anaemia should be excluded as contributory causes of symptoms.

Pruritus: The aetiology of pruritus in PBC is unclear. Fluctuations by day and over time are seen. Pruritus may lessen in end-stage liver disease. Cholestyramine (16 g/day 4 hours before UDCA) – a bile acid sequestrant – is commonly used in the treatment of pruritus, but is often poorly tolerated. Rifampicin, naltrexone (an opioid antagonist) or sertraline are alternatives. Gabapentin and cimetidine may also be effective.

Liver transplantation: Patients should be referred for transplant assessment once bilirubin is >103 μmol/L or MELD score is >12. Survival following transplantation is >80%.

Follow-up

• *Portal hypertension (PHT):* PHT can develop in pre-cirrhotic and cirrhotic patients. At the pre-cirrhotic stage the inflammatory reaction within the lobules causes obliteration of the portal venules leading to PHT. Variceal surveillance is recommended every 2–3 years.

• *Osteoporosis:* patients with PBC have an increased risk of osteoporosis. A DEXA scan is indicated at diagnosis and every 1–5 years. Calcium and vitamin D supplements should be prescribed for prophylaxis and bisphosphonates once osteoporosis is established. Hormone replacement therapy is also effective in post-menopausal women.

• Thyroid disease is a common association. Thyroid stimulating hormone should therefore be checked annually.

• *HCC surveillance:* 6-monthly AFP and US are recommended once cirrhotic and in older men with PBC.

• *Hyperlipidaemia:* serum lipids are often significantly elevated but probably only requires treatment if additional risk factors are present or there is a family history of cardiovascular disease.

• *Fat-soluble vitamin deficiencies:* decreased bile acid secretion can result in lipid malabsorption and fat-soluble vitamin (A, D, E, K) deficiencies. If the bilirubin remains elevated annual measurement of vitamin A, D and K is recommended and replacement provided as necessary.

• *Screening of family members:* PBC has a genetic predisposition and screening of female first-degree family members (alkaline phosphatase and AMA) should be considered, although benefit is uncertain.

Prognosis

PBC is a chronic progressive cholestatic disease that progresses over decades to end-stage liver disease. Median survival once symptomatic is 10–15 years but nowadays many cases are detected before symptoms arise and outlook is much improved with early treatment. Mayo and MELD scores are used to predict survival.

33 Sclerosing cholangiopathies

Box 33-1 Differential diagnosis of a biliary stricture

Choledocholithiasis/Mirizzi's syndrome
Chronic pancreatitis
Primary sclerosing cholangitis
Pancreatic cancer
Cholangiocarcinoma
Extraluminal compression (e.g. lymph nodes)
Postoperative (ischaemic, post-inflammatory)
Post-biliary sphincterotomy
Post-radiation therapy
Infective (TB, histoplasmosis, viral, parasitic, HIV cholangiopathy)
IgG4-related sclerosing cholangitits

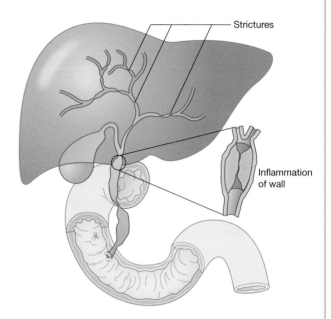

Figure 33-1 Primary sclerosing cholangitis (PSC).

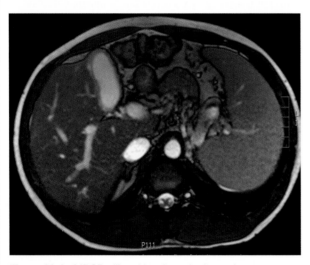

Figure 33-2 MRCP: dilated intrahepatic ducts above a hilar stricture.

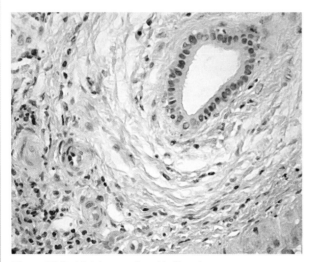

Figure 33-3 Histology: onion skin fibrosis.

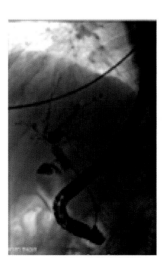

Figure 33-4 ERCP: multiple intrahepatic bile duct strictures and beading.

Hepatology at a Glance, First Edition. Deepak Joshi, Geri Keane and Alison Brind.
© 2015 John Wiley & Sons, Ltd. Published 2015 by John Wiley & Sons, Ltd. Companion website: www.ataglanceseries.com/hepatology

Primary sclerosing cholangitis

Primary sclerosing cholangitis (PSC) is a chronic cholestatic liver disease characterised by stricturing and dilatation of the intra- and extrahepatic bile ducts. **Small duct PSC** is a variant of PSC characterised by cholestatic biochemisty and histological features of PSC but with normal bile ducts on imaging (cholangiogram).

Epidemiology

PSC has an estimated prevalence of 6 cases per 100 000 population with a 2 : 1 male preponderance. The mean age of onset is 25–40 years. Approximately 60–80% of patients have concomitant inflammatory bowel disease (IBD; 87% will have ulcerative colitis and 13% Crohn's disease). Only 3–10% of patients with IBD develop PSC.

Pathogenesis

The aetiology of PSC is unknown but its pathogenesis is thought to be immune-mediated and it is associated with HLA-A1, -B8 and -DR3. PSC is characterised by biliary inflammation and fibrosis. Inflammation of the biliary epithelium causes necrosis and fibrous leading to duct and secondary parenchymal damage. PSC is a progressive disease that results in end-stage liver disease in most patients.

Clinical presentation

Common presenting features include jaundice, fatigue, pruritus and right upper quadrant pain. However, many cases are detected incidentally due to abnormal liver biochemistry. Features of cholangitis are rare prior to therapeutic interventions such as ERCP.

Investigations

Large duct PSC is diagnosed in patients with cholestatic LFTs and characteristic imaging. Other blood tests are of limited clinical use due to the wide range of autoantibody profiles that can be present; however, approximately 60% will have a raised serum IgG. MRCP is the imaging modality of choice in suspected PSC and typically demonstrates 'beading' (dilatation of the bile ducts proximal to a stricture). Imaging is also necessary to exclude secondary causes of sclerosing cholangitis and any complications of PSC. A liver biopsy is rarely necessary for diagnosis unless imaging is normal, raising the possibility of small duct PSC, or an overlap syndrome is suspected (e.g. disproportionately elevated transaminases). If undertaken, a liver biopsy will typically show ductopenia ('vanishing bile ducts'), concentric fibrosis of the intrahepatic ducts (onion skin pattern; Figure 33.3) and bile duct proliferation. However, none of these histological features are unique to PSC.

Management

Ursodeoxycholic acid: When this hydrophilic bile acid is given at moderate doses in PSC, liver function tests may improve. However, it has no effect on symptoms or overall survival and therefore is not prescribed routinely. Some studies suggest it may ameliorate against colorectal cancer risk.

Steroids and immunosuppressants: No role in classic PSC but may be beneficial in IgG4-related sclerosing cholangitis and overlap syndromes (see Chapter 34).

Cholestyramine: Used to manage associated pruritus. Rifampicin and naltrexone (an opioid antagonist) are alternatives if refractory.

Surgical and endoscopic biliary drainage: A dominant stricture is defined as a stricture with a diameter of ≤1.5 mm in diameter of the common bile duct and/or ≤1.0 mm of right or left hepatic ducts. It occurs in approximately half of PSC patients during follow-up and should always raise the suspicion of cholangiocarcinoma (CC). If patients develop jaundice or progressive worsening of their LFTs, endoscopic therapy (balloon dilatation of the stricture or stent placement) is recommended. Brush cytology should be obtained at the time of endotherapy to exclude malignancy. Injecting contrast into an obstructed system may introduce infection, leading to subsequent cholangitis. Therefore all patients with PSC undergoing an ERCP should receive prophylactic antibiotics. If the endoscopic approach is unsuccessful a percutaneous or surgical approach can be considered (see Chapter 8).

Nutrition: As in other cholestatic liver diseases, fat-soluble vitamin deficiencies should be corrected. Calcium and vitamin D are prescribed routinely to prevent osteopenia and bisphosphonates once osteoporosis is established.

Liver transplantation: Refractory pruritus, recurrent cholangitis, portal hypertension and/or decompensatation are indications for liver transplant assessment. Outcomes following transplant in PSC are superior to many other liver diseases with 80–90% 5-year survival; however, 25–30% develop recurrence of PSC in the graft at 5 years.

Complications

- *Portal hypertension (PHT):* PHT may occur in PSC prior to cirrhosis. At diagnosis approximately one-third of patients will have oesophageal varices.
- *Malignancy:* 7–9% of patients with PSC develop CC over a 10-year period. Colorectal cancer in more prevalent in patients with ulcerative colitis and PSC, annual surveillance colonoscopies are therefore advised.
- *Gallbladder disease:* 6–14% of patients with PSC develop gallbladder polyps of which up to half contain malignant cells on resection. An annual gallbladder US is therefore recommended and cholecystectomy once a gallbladder polyp is detected.
- *Overlap syndromes:* 1–17% of patients with PSC develop an overlap syndrome (see Chapter 34).

Prognosis

PSC is a progressive disease, with few effective medical treatments. Median survival from diagnosis to death or liver transplantation is 12–15 years. Small-duct PSC is associated with a better prognosis with fewer patients developing end-stage liver disease or CC.

Secondary sclerosing cholangitis

Secondary sclerosing cholangitis (SCC) is a stricturing disease, similar to PSC, which develops as a result of chronic biliary obstruction (e.g. choledocholithiasis or previous bile duct surgery).

IgG4-related sclerosing cholangitis

IgG4-related sclerosing cholangitis (IgG4-SC) is a further form of sclerosing cholangitis. Aetiology is unknown but it commonly affects middle-aged men. Imaging may resemble PSC or CC and it is characterised by a cholangiopathy with raised serum IgG4 levels (normal 8–140 mg/dL) and a lymphoplasmacytic infiltrate on biopsy. IgG4-SC is frequently associated with autoimmune pancreatitis and less commonly with sialadenitis and retroperitoneal fibrosis.

Management

IgG4-SC is primarily managed with corticosteroids, which leads to the resolution of clinical and radiological features of the disease. However, up to half of patients relapse following successful treatment and will therefore require a further course of steroids ± long-term immunosuppression. Long-term prognosis of the disease is unclear.

34 Overlap syndromes

	PBC	AIH	PSC	IgG4-SC
Common presenting features	Asymptomatic, jaundice fatigue, pruritis	Asymptomatic, transaminitis, jaundice, arthralgia	Asymptomatic, cholangitis, abdominal pain	Jaundice, fleeting, cholangiopathy, pancreatic mass
Autoimmune profile	Anti-mitochrondial antibody M2 (90–95%)	SMA (70–80%) LKM ANA (>1:40) and or pANCA (50–96%)	No definitive serum profile ANA (8–77%) SMA (0–83%) pANCA (26–94%)	Elevated IgG4 levels
Typical histology	Focal duct obliteration with granuloma 'florid duct lesion'	Portal mononuclear cell inflitration and interface hepatitis	Biliary changes – periductal sclerosis (onion skin lesions) Interface hepatitis and portal lymphocytic infiltration. All are variable findings	Periductal lymphoplasmacytic infiltrate with obliterative phlebitis and storiform fibrosis or lymphoplasmacytic infiltrate with storiform fibrosis and abundant IgG4 cells (>10 IgG4 cell/HPF)
		(a)		
Imaging	Normal or signs of liver cirrhosis	Normal or signs of liver cirrhosis	Cholangiopathy (with multiple strictures and beading) is characteristic. Not seen in small duct PSC	Cholangiopathy, 'sausage-shaped' pancreas and retroperitoneal fibrosis are characteristic. IgG4-SC can also be sub-divided based on the position of the stricture. Type 1, stenosis of the lower CBD type; type 2, intrahepatic stenosis with pre-stenotic dilatation; type 3, hilar and lower CBD stenosis; type 4; hilar stenosis only
Treatment	Consider UDCA: 10–15 mg/kg/day	Predisolone (30 mg/day) and azathioprine (1–2 mg/kg). Slowly taper steroids as transaminases normalise. Combination therapy for maintenance		Predisolone (20–40 mg/day). Continue until imaging and biochemistry improve. If patients relapse consider a further course of steroids ± long-term immuno-suppression with with azathioprine or rituximab
Other organs involved	Associated with other autoimmune disorders (e.g. Sjögren's syndrome, Hashimoto's thyroiditis, Sicca syndrome, CREST/Raynaud's phenomenon and coeliac disease (see Chapter 32)	Associated with other autoimmune disorders e.g. Hashimoto's thyroiditis, inflammatory bowel disease and diabetes	More than 80% have inflammatory bowel disease and of these 87% will have ulcerative colitis and 13% Crohn's disease	Multiorgan involment is common (e.g. autoimmune pancreatitis, sclerosing sialadenitis, retroperitoneal fibrosis and mediastinal lymphadenopathy)

(a) Source: *Mieli-Vergani, G. & Vergani, D. (2011)* Reproduced with permission of Nature Publishing Group.

Hepatology at a Glance, First Edition. Deepak Joshi, Geri Keane and Alison Brind.
© 2015 John Wiley & Sons, Ltd. Published 2015 by John Wiley & Sons, Ltd. Companion website: www.ataglanceseries.com/hepatology

Autoimmune hepatitis (AIH), primary biliary cirrhosis (PBC) and primary sclerosing cholangitis (PSC) are unique autoimmune liver diseases that share many of the same serological, biochemical, histological and aetiological features to differing extents.

When patients demonstrate features of more than one autoimmune liver disease simultaneously they are often said to have an overlap syndrome. Formal definitions for the overlap syndromes do not exist and the latest guidance from the International Autoimmune Hepatitis Group (IAIHG) suggests that patients with autoimmune liver disease should ideally be categorised by their predominant disease (e.g. AIH, PBC or PSC) rather than by one of the overlap syndromes. The rationale is that overlap features are often not sufficiently distinct or prevalent to become diagnostic entities in their own right.

However, since the term is still widely used in clinical practice some of the commonly described patterns of overlap, their recognisable features and management have been outlined here.

AIH–PBC

The prevalence of AIH–PBC overlap syndromes vary from 3% to 13% in patients initially diagnosed with AIH and 1–19% in those initially diagnosed with PBC.

AIH with PBC

Approximately 10% of patients with autoimmune hepatitis (AIH) will have a persistently elevated AMA. Without histological features of PBC (florid duct lesions and granulomas) these cases are not considered to be a true overlap syndrome but part of the spectrum of AIH. One-quarter of patients with overlap in AIH have a positive anti-smooth muscle antibody (ASMA). Often patients have features of both diseases from the outset. Less commonly patients with PBC may develop AIH during follow-up, sometimes many years after diagnosis.

PBC with subsequent AIH

This syndrome should be considered in PBC patients with persistently elevated transaminases. Interface or lobular hepatitis is present on biopsy. Use of the IAIHG score to diagnose AIH in overlap can be clinically useful but has not been validated for this indication.

Management

Patients often respond well to a combination of UCDA (12–15 mg/kg/day) with corticosteroids. Addition of azathioprine should be considered if AIH features predominate.

AIH–PSC

This syndrome is characterised by features of AIH (ANA, SMA, high titres of IgG and interface hepatitis) as well as overt cholangiographic or histological features of PSC. Approximately 7–14% of patients with AIH have imaging suggestive of PSC and 1–54% of patients with PSC will have feature of of AIH. It is more common in children and young adults diagnosed with AIH or PSC.

In AIH dominant disease, onset of overlap may be concurrent but often, the PSC component develops several years later. AIH–PSC overlap should always be considered in AIH patients who are poorly responsive to immunosuppressive therapy. An MRCP is highly recommended in children and young adults diagnosed with AIH to exclude concurrent PSC (recognising that imaging may be normal in the early stages of PSC.

Overlap in PSC dominant disease (autoimmune sclerosing cholangitis) is characterised by persistently elevated transaminases and autoimmune features (e.g. elevated ANA, SMA and IgG). A fall in transaminases in response to a trial of steroids is diagnostically useful, but confirmation of the presence of overlap is obtained through a liver biopsy.

Management

Requires a combination of UCDA, prednisolone and azathioprine. Biliary disease is progressive in approximately 50% but prognosis remains better than classic PSC.

PBC–PSC

Overlap between PBC and PSC has only been reported in a handful of cases. Histologically, these diseases can have similar appearances; however, typical cholangiographic features of large duct PSC with a positive AMA may suggest this syndrome.

AIH–Hepatitis C

Some patients with chronic hepatitis C demonstrate a positive autoimmune serological profile (positive anti-LKM-1, ANA, SMA, and a raised IgG) in addition to positive HCV serology (HCvAb and HCV RNA positivity). Histologically, they have features of AIH and HCV.

Management

Management of these patients can be particularly challenging as interferon may worsen AIH, while any immunosuppression for AIH may increase HCV replication. Presence of LKM-1 antibody is suggestive of dominant HCV hepatitis; typically these patients lack antibodies to cytochrome P-450 and generally they respond well to standard AIH treatment with interferon.

Haemochromatosis and iron overload

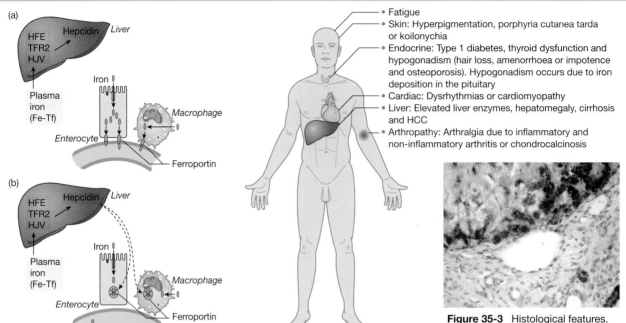

Figure 35-1 Pathophysiology of iron absorption.
(a) iron deficiency; (b) iron excess.
Source: Utzschneider, K.M. & Kowdley, K.V. (2010).
Reproduced with permission of Nature Publishing Group.

- Fatigue
- Skin: Hyperpigmentation, porphyria cutanea tarda or koilonychia
- Endocrine: Type 1 diabetes, thyroid dysfunction and hypogonadism (hair loss, amenorrhoea or impotence and osteoporosis). Hypogonadism occurs due to iron deposition in the pituitary
- Cardiac: Dysrhythmias or cardiomyopathy
- Liver: Elevated liver enzymes, hepatomegaly, cirrhosis and HCC
- Arthropathy: Arthralgia due to inflammatory and non-inflammatory arthritis or chondrocalcinosis

Figure 35-2 Complications of haemochromatosis.

Figure 35-3 Histological features. Marked iron deposition – confirmed with Perls' reagent.

Table 35-1 Clinical phenotypes of hereditary haemochromatosis (HH).

Genetic abnormality	Person affected	Predominant clinical features
HFE	Middle aged, white northern European male	Fatigue, bronzed skin, arthralgia and hepatomegaly, familial
TfR2	Any race, male or female, age 30–40	Cardiomyopathy, diabetes, liver disease
HJV or HAMP	Any race, male or female, age 15–20	Cardiomyopathy, impotence or amenorrhoea
FPN	Any race, male or female, any age	Familial

Table 35-2 Investigations in HH.

Test	Comments
Serum ferritin	Serum ferritin estimates total body iron stores. Levels >300 µg/L in men and post-menopausal women and >200 µg/L in younger women is suggestive in HH. However, ferritin is an acute phase protein and can be elevated for many reasons (e.g. chronic alcohol consumption, inflammation, sepsis). In early HH, serum ferritin may also be normal
Transferritin saturation (TS)	TS indicates the amount of iron that is readily available for use. The average is 30%. If it is persistently >50% in men or >45% in women, HH is likely
Liver function tests	Elevated liver enzymes occur in one-third of patients with HH, 6% of men and 2% of women will have cirrhosis
HFE genetic test	HFE gene testing should be performed in all patients with unexplained chronic liver disease and a raised TS. Consideration should be given to testing those with porphyria cutanea tarda, well-defined chondrocalcinosis, type 1 diabetes and HCC without a clear risk factor
Cardiac investigations	Echocardiogram and increasingly cardiac MR are used to diagnosis cardiac iron deposition and/or cardiomyopathy
Liver MR	MR can be used to estimate hepatic iron concentration
Liver biopsy	With the introduction of HFE mutation analysis a liver biopsy is rarely required for the diagnosis of HH. However, it remains an invaluable test when the diagnosis remains uncertain or the staging of liver disease is deemed necessary

Causes of iron overload

Hereditary haemochromatosis (HH):
* *HFE*-related HH (90%);
* Non-*HFE*-related HH (10%).

Secondary iron overload:
* Iron-loading anaemias (e.g. thalassemia major, sideroblastic, aplastic anaemia, red cell aplasia and sickle cell anaemia);
* Parenteral iron overload (e.g. multiple blood transfusions);
* Chronic liver disease: ALD, hepatitis B or C, NAFLD.

Hereditary haemochromatosis

HH is genetic disorder of unregulated iron absorption, leading to a state of iron overload. Excess iron is deposited in organs, such as the liver, pancreas, pituitary, skin and joints, which over many years leads to organ damage and dysfunction. The highest incidence of HH worldwide is seen in Ireland. It is infrequently encountered in southern Europe, Africa and Asia.

Genetics

HH is the most common inherited disorder in the Caucasian population. The majority of cases arise as a result of a missense mutation of the *HFE* gene (situated on chromosome 6). The missense mutation C282Y is responsible for the majority of cases of HH. *HFE* C282Y homozygosity is present in 80% of patients with clinical iron overload and up to 90% of patients with HH. However, <15% of C282Y homozygotes in the general population develop clinically symptomatic iron overload. This discrepancy is likely to be due to undefined, genetic and/or environmental factors. Homozygosity for H63D (an alternative *HFE* mutation) and heterozygous mutations for C282Y or H63D may result in an increased ferritin and/or transferrin saturation but rarely are sufficient to cause iron overload.

In the 10% of patients with HH without an *HFE* mutation clinical iron overload may result from mutations in the transmembrane iron transporter ferroportin (*FPN*), haemojuvelin (*HJV*), transferrin receptor 2 (*TfR2*) or the hepcidin gene (*HAMP*). Each mutation results in a slightly different clinical phenotype (Table 35.1).

Population screening for HH is not recommended due to the low penetrance of *HFE* genes. Screening of first-degree relatives and those with an appropriate clinical phenotype is advisable.

Pathogenesis

Iron absorption occurs primarily in the duodenum and jejunum. Genes associated with HH control iron homeostasis. Hepcidin is a circulating antimicrobial peptide that is secreted from the liver and is responsible for regulating iron transportation at a cellular level. In states of iron deficiency, hepcidin levels are low and the iron transport protein ferroportin allows iron to pass from duodenal enterocytes into the blood and from macrophages into the plasma. When excess iron is present, hepcidin levels increase, ferroportin undergoes degradation and iron absorption from the gut decreases. Mutations in the *HFE* gene results in low hepcidin levels, so the enterocytes act like they are in an iron deficient state and despite high circulating levels of iron, absorption of iron by the enterocyte continues (Figure 35.1).

Clinical presentation

The classic triad of 'bronze skin', diabetes and cirrhosis occurs in less than 8% of cases. Up to half of patients with HH are completely asymptomatic and are diagnosed as a result of an incidental finding of a raised ferritin or familial screening. Other associated features include:
* *Fatigue*;
* *Skin*: hyperpigmentation, porphyria cutanea tarda or koilonychias;
* *Arthropathy*: arthralgia due to inflammatory and non-inflammatory arthritis or chondrocalcinosis;
* *Endocrine*: type 1 diabetes, thyroid dysfunction and hypogonadism (hair loss, amenorrhoea or impotence and osteoporosis). Hypogonadism occurs due to iron deposition in the pituitary;
* *Cardiac*: dysrhythmias or cardiomyopathy;
* *Liver*: abnormal LFTs, hepatomegaly, cirrhosis and HCC.

Investigations

See Table 35.2.

Treatment

The overall aim of treatment in HH is to reduce serum iron levels. This is achieved by:
* *Venesection*: initially performed weekly. Each pint of blood removed contains 200 mg iron. Post-venesection the body uses the excess stored iron to make new red blood cells, therefore reducing the overall iron load. Venesection should continue until iron levels are satisfactory, which may take several months. During this period the haemoglobin is monitored weekly and iron indices every few weeks. Once the serum ferritin is below 50 µg/L, maintenance venesections can be performed with a target serum ferritin of 50–100 µg/L, usually every few months.
* *Chelation* (e.g. desferrioxamine): in patients with comorbidities or who have poor venous access, iron chelating agents are an alternative to venesection.
* Patients should be advised to minimise alcohol intake; cirrhosis is nine times more common in patients with HH who drink >6 units/day.
* *HCC surveillance*: 6-monthly surveillance US scans are recommended once patients become cirrhotic. Up to one-third of HH deaths are thought to be due to HCC.
* *Screening*: offer genetic screening to first-degree relatives.
* *Surgery*: liver transplantation is occasionally indicated in those who develop end-stage liver failure. In HH 5-year survival post-transplantation is lower than many other indications (<50%), largely due to septic and cardiac complications.

Prognosis

Early diagnosis and treatment in HH is crucial. However, a normal lifespan can be expected if treatment is commenced before liver and diabetic complications have developed.

36 Wilson's disease

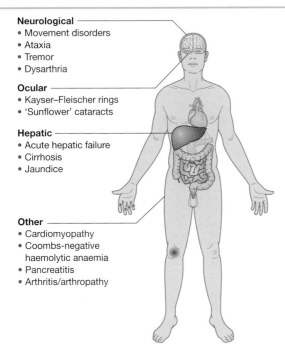

Neurological
- Movement disorders
- Ataxia
- Tremor
- Dysarthria

Ocular
- Kayser–Fleischer rings
- 'Sunflower' cataracts

Hepatic
- Acute hepatic failure
- Cirrhosis
- Jaundice

Other
- Cardiomyopathy
- Coombs-negative haemolytic anaemia
- Pancreatitis
- Arthritis/arthropathy

Figure 36-1 Features of Wilson's disease.

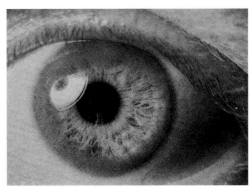

Figure 36-2 Kayser–Fleischer ring – brown deposit at the periphery of the cornea.

Source: *Dooley JS et al. (eds) Sherlock's Diseases of the Liver and Biliary System, 12th Edition (2011). Reproduced with permission of John Wiley & Sons Ltd.*

Wilson's disease

An autosomal recessive disorder that leads to impaired cellular transport of copper and accumulation in the liver, brain and cornea. Affects 1 in 30 000 live births. Occurs due to mutations of the *ATP7B* gene on chromosome 13. Variable clinical penetrance with presentation in childhood or adulthood. Majority of patients present between the ages of 5 and 35 years. However, the diagnosis of Wilson's disease should be considered in any patient with liver abnormalities and neurological disorder.

Clinical presentation

Manifestations are usually hepatic, neurologic and psychiatric, with most patients presenting with a combination of symptoms. Regardless of clinical presentation, patients often develop other organ involvement as the disease progresses.

Hepatic
- Asymptomatic abnormal liver biochemistry;
- Acute or chronic hepatitis;
- Jaundice;
- Steatosis;
- Acute liver failure; associated with Coombs-negative haemolytic anaemia;
- Compensated or decompensated cirrhosis.

Ocular
- Kayser–Fleischer (KF) rings (brown–grey in colour) are due to copper deposition in Desçemet's membrane in the periphery of the cornea. This is the clinical hallmark of Wilson's disease occurring in 95% patients but its absence does not exclude the disease as it is present in 50% of patients with hepatic disease. Often only detected by slit-lamp examination.
- Copper can also be deposited in the lens and present as sunflower cataracts.

Neurological
Nearly all patients (98%) with neurological manifestations will have KF rings. Presentation can be divided into the following catorgories:
- Dysarthria: most common neurologic symptom (85–97% of patients);
- Gait abnormalities/ataxia;
- Dystonia;
- Tremor: resting or with action, can be asymmetrical;
- Parkinsonism;
- Seizures;
- Autonomic dysfunction.

Patients can also present with cognitive impairment and dementia as well as behavioural and psychiatric symptoms including acute psychosis. MR and CT imaging of the brain can identify areas of copper deposition. Involvement of the basal ganglia, thalamus and brainstem is suggestive of Wilson's disease. Cerebrospinal fluid sampling is rarely required but if performed will demonstrate elevated copper levels.

Other

Copper can also be deposited in other organs. Less common manifestations include:

- Cardiomyopathy;
- Haemolysis: Coombs-negative haemolytic anaemia;
- Pancreatitis;
- Arthritis/arthropathy;
- Fanconi's syndrome (glycosuria, amino-aciduria, hypouricaemia and proximal renal tubular acidosis);
- Nephrolithiasis.

Diagnosis

Wilson's disease should be considered in any patient with unexplained liver, neurologic or psychiatric symptoms.

- Slit-lamp examination: examine for KF rings.
- Serum ceruloplasmin: decreased by 50% but can be normal.
- Serum copper: low. Can be high in patients with cholestasis.
- 24-hour urinary copper: >1.6 µmol/24 hours. Can be high in patients with an acute hepatitis or with cholestasis. Raised by penicillamine in affected patients more than carriers.
- Liver biopsy: parenchymal copper >4 µmol/g dry weight. Changes include steatosis to macronodular cirrhosis.
- Mutation analysis: whole gene sequencing is possible. Recommended for screening first-degree relatives of patients with Wilson's disease.

Making the diagnosis of Wilson's disease can be difficult. The Wilson's disease scoring system can help improve the diagnostic certainty (Table 36.1).

Prognosis

Untreated, Wilson's disease is fatal and treatment is therefore lifelong. Progression is usually gradual but sudden deteriorations can occur. Most patients will die from the hepatic manifestations.

Treatment

Neurological symptoms can worsen after beginning treatment.

D-penicillamine: Promotes urinary excretion of copper and induces metallothionein (endogenous chelator of metals). Usually taken 1–2 hours before meals to inhibit dietary absorption of copper. Adequacy of treatment can be monitored by performing 24-hour urinary copper excretion. Goal of therapy is to increase urinary copper excretion from baseline levels and a normal serum copper.

Trientine: Chelates copper and then promotes urinary copper excretion. Associated with iron deficiency. Fewer side effects than D-penicillamine.

Zinc: Reduces uptake of copper from the gastrointestinal tract and induces metallothionein in enterocytes. Bound copper is then excreted faecally.

Liver transplantation: Medical therapy is rarely effective in patients with acute liver failure. A prognostic score (Table 36.2) ≥11 is fatal without liver transplantation. Defect is corrected with transplantation.

Table 36.1 Wilson's scoring system

Typical clinical symptoms and signs		Other investigations	
KF rings		**Liver copper (in the absence of cholestasis)**	
Present	2	>5 × ULN (>4 µmol/g)	2
Absent	0	0.8–4.0 µmol/g	1
		Normal (<0.8 µmol/g)	–1
		Rhodanine-positive granules[a]	1
Neurological symptoms[b]		**Urinary copper (acute hepatitis having been excluded)**	
Severe	2	Normal	0
Mild	1	1–2 × ULN	1
Absent	0	>2 × ULN	2
		Normal, but >5 × ULN after D-pencillamine	2
Serum caeruloplasmin		**Mutation analysis**	
Normal (>0.2 g/L)	0	On both chromosomes detected	4
0.1–0.2 g/L	1	On 1 chromosome detected	1
<0.1 g/L	2	No mutations detected	0
Coombs-negative haemolytic anaemia			
Present	1		
Absent	0		
TOTAL SCORE		**INTERPRETATION**	
≥4		Diagnosis established	
3		Possible diagnosis, more tests required	
≤2		Diagnosis unlikely	

[a]If quantitative liver copper unavailable.
[b]Or typical abnormalities at brain MRI.

Table 36.2 Prognostic index in Wilson's disease

	1	2	3	4
Serum bilirubin (µmol/L)	100–150	151–200	201–300	>300
AST (U/L)	100–150	151–300	301–400	>400
INR	1.3–1.6	1.7–1.9	2.0–2.4	>2.4
WBC (10^9/L)	6.8–8.3	8.4–10.3	10.4–15.3	>15.3
Albumin (g/L)	34–44	25–33	21–24	<21

37 Metabolic disorders

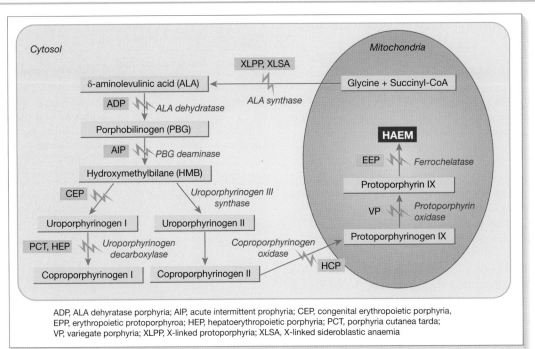

ADP, ALA dehyratase porphyria; AIP, acute intermittent prophyria; CEP, congenital erythropoietic porphyria, EPP, erythropoietic protoporphyroa; HEP, hepatoerythropoietic porphyria; PCT, porphyria cutanea tarda; VP, variegate porphyria; XLPP, X-linked protoporphyria; XLSA, X-linked sideroblastic anaemia

GSD type	Enzyme deficiency	Eponym	Clinical features	Treatment
Oa	Glycogen synthase-2	–	Ketotic hypoglycaemia, no hepatomegaly	Uncooked cornstarch
I	Glucose-6-phosphatase	Von Gierke's disease	Ketotic hypoglycaemia, hepatomegaly, lactic acidosis, hyperuricaemia, hyperlipidaemia, hypertriglyceridaemia, neutropenia	Uncooked cornstarch, allopurinol, GCSF
III	Glycogen debrancher	Cori's disease or Forbes' disease	Ketosis, hypoglycaemia, hepatomegaly	Uncooked starch
IV	Glycogen branching	Andersen disease	Hepatomegaly	Liver transplantation
VI	Liver phosphorylase	Hers' disease	Hepatomegaly, mild hypoglycaemia	No specific treatment
IXa	Phosphorylase kinase	–	Hepatomegaly, mild hypoglycaemia, fatigue	No specific treatment
	Glucose transporter 2 (GLUT2)	Fanconi–Bickel syndrome	Growth retardation, Fanconi syndrome, galactosaemia	Small meals, cornstarch

Hepatology at a Glance, First Edition. Deepak Joshi, Geri Keane and Alison Brind.
© 2015 John Wiley & Sons, Ltd. Published 2015 by John Wiley & Sons, Ltd. Companion website: www.ataglanceseries.com/hepatology

Metabolic disorders

Inborn errors of metabolism are rare. Neurologic and gastrointestinal features are common. Neurologic manifestations include lethargy, coma, development delay, ataxia and weakness. Jaundice, hepato-splenomagly, vomiting and diarrhoea are the common gastrointestinal manifestations. Biochemical abnormalities include lactic acidosis, hyperammonaemia, hypoglycaemia, pancytopenia and raised transaminases.

Porphyrias

The porphyrias occur secondary to defects in the enzymes involved in haem biosynthesis pathway. The majority of haem synthesis occurs in the bone marrow (erythropoietic) while the remaining occurs in the liver (hepatic) primarily for the production of various cytochrome P450 (CYP450) enzymes.

Acute intermittent porphyria

This occurs due to a partial deficiency in porphobilinogen (PBG) deaminase. Autosomal dominance inheritance. Presents with non-specific symptoms (abdominal pain, neuro/psychiatric symptoms) and red–brown urine.

Triggers: Any drug that induces CP450, progesterone, fasting, stress.

Diagnosis: Increased urinary aminolevulinic acid and PBG.

Treatment: Avoid drugs known to be contraindicated (check with www.porphyriafoundation.com). Intravenous glucose loading or use of intravenous haemin. Liver transplantation maybe indicated in patients with severe recurrent episodes. Patients over 50 years of age require annual screening for HCC.

Porphyria cutanea tarda

This is the most common porphyria and occurs due to a deficiency of hepatic uroporphyrinogen decarboxylase. Can be sporadic (type I) or familial (type II). Similar enzyme defect also occurs in hepatoerythropoietic porphyria.

Porphyria cutanea tarda is an iron dependent disease which usually presents in mid or late adulthood. Classic presentation is with a blistering skin rash or hyperpigmentation in sun-exposed areas. Raised ALT/AST is common. Liver injury occurs partly due accumulation of porphyrins. Increased susceptibility is recognised in patients with iron overload, alcohol excess, smokers, HCV infection, HIV infection and use of the OCP.

Diagnosis: Increased plasma or urinary porphyrins.

Treatment: Skin protection; phlebotomy to reduce serum ferritin or low dose hydroxychloroquine.

Glycogen storage disease

Occurs due to defects in glycogen synthesis or breakdown within the liver, muscles and other cells. Fifteen types of glycogen storage disease have been identified. Patients usually present in infancy or childhood with hypoglycaemia, ketosis, hepatomegaly and lactic acidosis. The table summarises the glycogen storage diseases associated with liver disease.

Lysosomal storage disorders

Occur due to defective lysosomal metabolism, defective cellular function or transport which results in the accumulation of glycoproteins, mucopolysaccharides or glycolipids within lysosomes. Presentation is usually in infancy and with hepatomegaly, splenomegaly and features of failing to thrive.

Fabry's disease

Also known as Anderson–Fabry disease. It is a X-linked inborn error of glycosphingolipid. The metabolic defect is deficiency or defect in the lysosomal hydrolase alpha-galactosidase resulting in the accumulation of globotriasylceramide within lysosomes in renal tubular and interstitial cells, cardiac muscle cells, vascular smooth muscle cells. Renal manifestations affect approximately 50% of patients by 35 years of age. Fabry's disease should be considered in patients with severe pain in the extremities, cutaneous vascular lesions, hypohidrosis and chronic kidney disease without a clear causative aetiology.

Gaucher's disease

The most common lysosomal storage disease. Highly prevalent in patients of Ashkenazi Jewish descent. An autosomal recessive disorder caused by a mutation in the glucocerebrosidase gene (found on chromosome 1q21). Occurs due to a deficiency of a lysosomal enzyme glucoysl-ceramide-β-glucosidase in leucocytes, hepatocytes and aminocytes. Three clinical subtypes exist (I–III). Type I is distinguished from types II and III by the lack of characteristic central nervous involvement. Diagnosis is made by demonstrating reduced enzyme activity in peripheral leucocytes. Treatment is by replacement of the deficient enzyme.

Hurler's syndrome

Hurler's syndrome is the severe form of type I mucopolysaccharides. Also known as gargoylism. It is characterised by the deficiency of α-L-iduronidase. Clinical features include skeletal abnormalities, hepatosplenomegaly and intellectual disability. Coarse facial features are also prominent as well as a widened nasal bridge and flattened mid face. Presentation is usually at 6–24 months. Investigations include measurement of urinary glycosaminoglycan concentration. To make a definitive diagnosis an assay of enzyme activity is required from peripheral blood leucocytes.

Familial hypercholestrolaemia

Autosomal disease due to the absence of the gene that encodes for the LDL receptor. Total cholesterol and LDL are increased. Xanthomas are present. Treatment is with reduction in dietary fats and introduction of bile acid sequestrants (i.e. cholestyramine and statins).

38 Multisystemic diseases

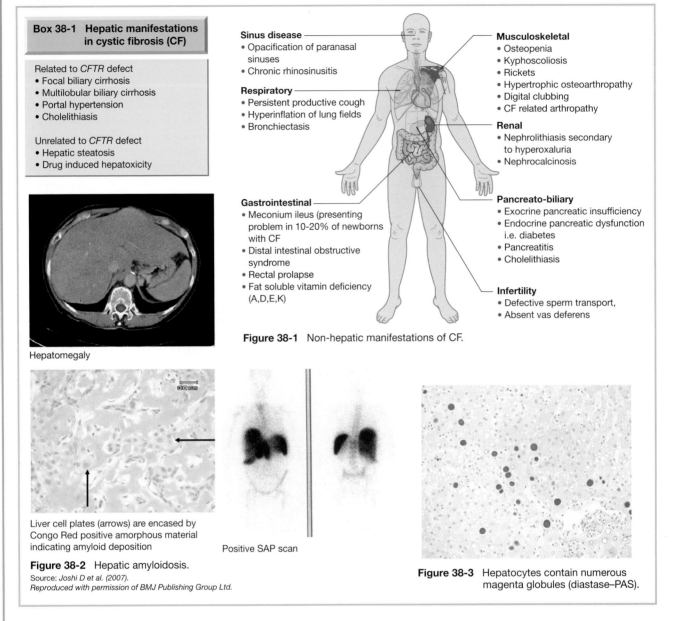

Box 38-1 Hepatic manifestations in cystic fibrosis (CF)

Related to *CFTR* defect
- Focal biliary cirrhosis
- Multilobular biliary cirrhosis
- Portal hypertension
- Cholelithiasis

Unrelated to *CFTR* defect
- Hepatic steatosis
- Drug induced hepatoxicity

Hepatomegaly

Sinus disease
- Opacification of paranasal sinuses
- Chronic rhinosinusitis

Respiratory
- Persistent productive cough
- Hyperinflation of lung fields
- Bronchiectasis

Gastrointestinal
- Meconium ileus (presenting problem in 10-20% of newborns with CF)
- Distal intestinal obstructive syndrome
- Rectal prolapse
- Fat soluble vitamin deficiency (A,D,E,K)

Musculoskeletal
- Osteopenia
- Kyphoscoliosis
- Rickets
- Hypertrophic osteoarthropathy
- Digital clubbing
- CF related arthropathy

Renal
- Nephrolithiasis secondary to hyperoxaluria
- Nephrocalcinosis

Pancreato-biliary
- Exocrine pancreatic insufficiency
- Endocrine pancreatic dysfunction i.e. diabetes
- Pancreatitis
- Cholelithiasis

Infertility
- Defective sperm transport,
- Absent vas deferens

Figure 38-1 Non-hepatic manifestations of CF.

Liver cell plates (arrows) are encased by Congo Red positive amorphous material indicating amyloid deposition

Figure 38-2 Hepatic amyloidosis.
Source: *Joshi D et al. (2007).*
Reproduced with permission of BMJ Publishing Group Ltd.

Positive SAP scan

Figure 38-3 Hepatocytes contain numerous magenta globules (diastase–PAS).

Cystic fibrosis

Cystic fibrosis (CF) is caused by a mutation in a gene on chromosome 7 encoding the cystic fibrosis transmembrane conductance regulator (CFTR) protein. The CFTR is a cyclic adenosine monophosphate (cAMP)-regulated epithelial chloride channel that can alter the activity of ionic transporters. Over 800 mutations in *CFTR* gene have been discovered but the most common is a base pair deletion in position 508 (ΔF508). Dysfunction of the CFTR protein causes impaired epithelial chloride, sodium and water transfer and results in increased mucus viscosity.

CF is the most common autosomal recessive disease amongst Caucasians, affecting 1 in 2000 live births. CF commonly affects the lungs, pancreas, sweat glands and gastrointestinal tract. Liver and hepatobiliary disease is becoming more common due to increased life expectancy. Severe liver disease is usually diagnosed before the second decade of life. CF-related liver disease (CFLD) is the third leading cause of death after respiratory and transplant-related complications.

The CFTR protein is located on the apical surface of intrahepatic and extrahepatic cholangiocytes. Dysfunction of the CFTR protein leads to thick viscous bile. Hepatic manifestations can be related or unrelated to the underlying *CFTR* defect.

Focal biliary cirrhosis: Pathognomic feature of CFLD and related to the *CFTR* defect in cholangiocytes. Results in biliary obstruction, toxic retention and progressive peri-portal fibrosis. May lead to multilobular cirrhosis and complications of portal hypertension.

Hepatic steatosis: Most common form of presentation. Likely related to nutritional state and fatty acid, carnitine and choline deficiencies.

Hepatology at a Glance, First Edition. Deepak Joshi, Geri Keane and Alison Brind.

Diagnosis

Liver disease maybe asymptomatic. A high index of suspicion for CFLD is required. Hepatomegaly is a common clinical presentation and may result from fatty infiltration or focal biliary cirrhosis. Abnormal LFTs maybe present (↑ ALP, ↑ AST/ALT, ↑ GGT). Abdominal US may identify hepatic steatosis or hepato-splenomegaly. Liver biopsy remains the gold standard for diagnosing but is not always necessary to diagnose CFLD.

Management

Optimisation of nutritional status, replacement of fat-soluble vitamins, carnitine and choline. Ursodeoxcholic acid (UDCA) is recommended (20 mg/kg/day) and may help increase bile flow and improve LFTs. Patients with portal hypertension should be managed with conventional methods. Liver transplantation is an option.

Sarcoidosis

Sarcoidosis is a multisystemic granulomatous disease of unknown aetiology, characterised by non-caseating epitheloid granulomas. Pulmonary involvement is common (90% of patients), the classic presentation being with bilateral hilar lymphadenopathy. The liver is the third most common organ where sarcoidosis is found but patients may be asymptomatic with mild abnormality in LFTs only (↑ ALP, ↑ GGT). Cirrhosis is a rare occurrence. Portal hypertension can occur due to peri-portal granulomas. Granulomas can also lead to hepatic vein obstruction. The diagnosis of hepatic sarcoid is confirmed on liver biopsy by demonstrating granulomas in the majority of the specimen, predominately in the portal tracts. Patients with severe cholestasis, intrahepatic biliary strictures and portal hypertension may benefit from a trial of corticosteroids. UDCA can also be used and may be of benefit.

Amyloidosis

Amyloidosis refers to a spectrum of diseases characterised by the deposition of fibrils in extracellular tissue. An insoluble matrix (resistant to proteolysis) is formed, the result of abnormal folding of circulating proteins. There are two major types: AL (primary), related to plasma cell dyscrasias, and AA (secondary), associated with chronic inflammatory disorders. Familial amyloidosis is an autosomal dominant disorder commonly caused by a mutation in transthyretin.

Amyloid can be deposited anywhere in the body (kidneys, liver, heart, gastrointestinal tract, peripheral nerves) except for the central nervous system. Organ dysfunction occurs once a critical amount of normal tissue is replaced by amyloid. Characteristic histological findings are a waxy amorphous material displaying the classic apple green birefringence under polarised light microscopy with Congo red staining. Intravenous injection of technetium labelled serum amyloid P component is both sensitive and specific for evidence of tissue amyloidosis deposits.

Hepatic involvement is common in both AL and AA amyloidosis. ALP is commonly raised. Clinical features include hepatomegaly and hyposplenism. Liver is classically described as 'rock-hard' on palpation. Stigmata of CLD are rare. Patients can present with cholestatic jaundice, ascites and fulminant hepatic failure. Liver biopsy is associated with an increased risk of bleeding (secondary to factor X deficiency and amyloid infiltration of vessels) and, rarely, hepatic rupture. Treatment is of the underlying disorder and complications of hepatic involvement (e.g. treatment of ascites).

α1-Antitrypsin deficiency

α1-Antitrypsin deficiency (A1AT) is a serine protease inhibitor produced by hepatocytes that inhibits neutrophil proteases. A1AT deficiency is associated with pulmonary, liver and skin disease. Normal levels of A1AT are seen in patients who carry the common allele (M) of the *A1AT* gene while the Z allele is the most deficient variant. A1AT deficiency is an autosomal dominant disease that can cause cirrhosis and HCC. The most common form of A1AT deficiency (PI*ZZ) occurs in patients who carry a homozygous variant of the *A1AT* gene (*SERPINA1*). Hepatic disease occurs due to the polymerisation and accumulation of the Z variant of *A1AT* in the endoplasmic reticulum, within hepatocytes. A1AT within hepatocytes stains positively with periodic acid–Schiff (PAS) reagent (see opposite). Diagnosis is made by the measurement of serum A1AT and genotyping of *A1AT* gene to detect the Z allele. No specific therapy is available but smoking should be avoided. Liver transplantation is an option.

PI*ZZ phenotype

Affects approximately 1 in 1600 births. Classically associated with lung disease (panacinar emphysema) and with a necrotising paniculitis. Pathogenesis of lung disease is due to an imbalance between neutrophil elastase, which destroys elastin, and the elastin inhibitor A1AT, which protects against proteolytic degradation of elastin.

- 10% of children develop neonatal cholestatic hepatitis the prognosis of which varies: 25% had no disease symptoms at the age of 10 but 25% needed a liver transplant at some point in childhood.
- 40% of adults have histological evidence of liver disease and cirrhosis. Male gender and obesity are risk factors for progression of liver disease.

PI*MZ phenotype

PI*MZ phenotype is associated with an increased risk of cirrhosis.

Heridatory haemorrhagic telangiectasia

Also known as Rendu–Osler–Weber disease. Rare (1–2 cases per 10 000 population) autosomal dominant disorder. Characterised by numerous arteriovenous malformations affecting the skin, lung, brain and/or liver. Defect thought to be related to the vascular endothelium. Common clinical presentations include high-output heart failure, portal hypertension and biliary ischaemia. Treatment depends on presentation.

39 Vascular disorders

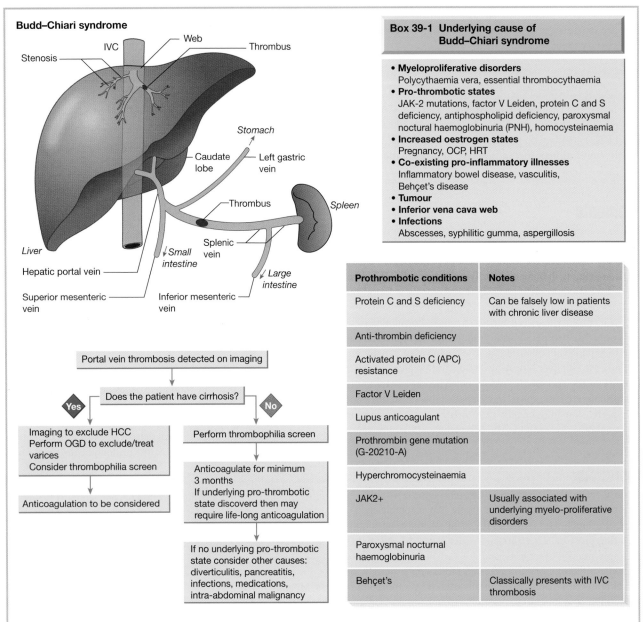

Budd–Chiari syndrome

Labels: Stenosis, IVC, Web, Thrombus, Stomach, Caudate lobe, Left gastric vein, Thrombus, Spleen, Liver, Small intestine, Splenic vein, Hepatic portal vein, Large intestine, Superior mesenteric vein, Inferior mesenteric vein

Portal vein thrombosis detected on imaging
→ Does the patient have cirrhosis?

Yes →
Imaging to exclude HCC
Perform OGD to exclude/treat varices
Consider thrombophilia screen
→ Anticoagulation to be considered

No →
Perform thrombophilia screen
→ Anticoagulate for minimum 3 months
If underlying pro-thrombotic state discoverd then may require life-long anticoagulation
→ If no underlying pro-thrombotic state consider other causes: diverticulitis, pancreatitis, infections, medications, intra-abdominal malignancy

Box 39-1 Underlying cause of Budd–Chiari syndrome

- **Myeloproliferative disorders**
  Polycythaemia vera, essential thrombocythaemia
- **Pro-thrombotic states**
  JAK-2 mutations, factor V Leiden, protein C and S deficiency, antiphospholipid deficiency, paroxysmal nocturnal haemoglobinuria (PNH), homocysteinaemia
- **Increased oestrogen states**
  Pregnancy, OCP, HRT
- **Co-existing pro-inflammatory illnesses**
  Inflammatory bowel disease, vasculitis, Behçet's disease
- **Tumour**
- **Inferior vena cava web**
- **Infections**
  Abscesses, syphilitic gumma, aspergillosis

Prothrombotic conditions	Notes
Protein C and S deficiency	Can be falsely low in patients with chronic liver disease
Anti-thrombin deficiency	
Activated protein C (APC) resistance	
Factor V Leiden	
Lupus anticoagulant	
Prothrombin gene mutation (G-20210-A)	
Hyperchromocysteinaemia	
JAK2+	Usually associated with underlying myelo-proliferative disorders
Paroxysmal nocturnal haemoglobinuria	
Behçet's	Classically presents with IVC thrombosis

Vascular disorders
Budd–Chiari syndrome

Budd–Chiari syndrome is characterised by obstruction of the hepatic veins or supra-hepatic vena cava. More common in women, it usually presents in the third or fourth decade but can occur in any age group. Clinical presentation can be with hepatic failure (acute), subacute or chronic. Right upper quadrant pain, hepatomegaly and ascites is the classic clinical presentation. Jaundice may not be present initially, but can develop rapidly.

Aetiology

Budd–Chiari syndrome can be divided into 'primary' causes (i.e. related to a thrombosis) or 'secondary' (i.e. related to compression or invasion of a lesion outside the vein). An underlying cause is identified in the majority of patients (see Box 39.1), the most common being an underlying myeloproliferative disorder. *JAK2* (Janus kinase 2) tyrosine kinase mutations are common in patients with Budd–Chiari syndrome, affecting up to 80%.

Hepatology at a Glance, First Edition. Deepak Joshi, Geri Keane and Alison Brind.
© 2015 John Wiley & Sons, Ltd. Published 2015 by John Wiley & Sons, Ltd. Companion website: www.ataglanceseries.com/hepatology

Diagnosis

Budd–Chiari syndrome should be considered in all patients with:
- Acute/chronic liver illness + ascites, abdominal pain or hepatomegaly;
- Liver disease in a patient with known risk factors for thrombosis.

An underlying cause should be sought in all patients. US, CT or MRI can aid the diagnosis. Caudate lobe hypertrophy is seen in 75% of patients due to direct drainage of this segment of liver directly into the IVC. Ascitic analysis typically demonstrates a high serum albumin–ascites gradient. A liver biopsy is usually not required but can be obtained at the time of a TIPS and can help establish whether there is cirrhosis.

Treatment

The underlying cause should be treated. Patients with fulminant hepatic failure (FHF) may require liver transplantation. The oral contraceptive pill (OCP) should be avoided. Subacute or chronic presentation should be managed firstly with anticoagulation which should be lifelong (to prevent propagation of the thrombosis) and diuretics to treat ascites. Thrombolytic agents are not usually recommended. Shunts may be required by:
- *Transjugular intrahepatic portosystemic shunt (TIPS):* creates an alternative venous outflow tract and decompresses congested segments. Complications include occlusion;
- *Surgery and liver transplantation:* surgical shunts (side-to-side portacaval, splenorenal) restore hepatic venous drainage but are only possible if the IVC is patent. Liver transplantation is indicated in patients with failed TIPS, FHF or progressive liver dysfunction.

Portal vein thrombosis

Can occur in patients with or without cirrhosis. An underlying pro-thrombotic state should be excluded in all patients. US with Doppler evaluation is recommended. A CT scan without contrast can demonstrate hyper-attenuating material within the vessel. CT is recommended to assess for thrombus extension. Spontaneous recanalisation can occur but is rare.

Acute presentation: Asymptomatic to abdominal pain, life threatening variceal bleeding or bowel infarction. Ascites is rare.

Chronic presentation: Also known as portal cavernoma. Usually with ascites or incidental finding on imaging. Can also present with variceal bleeding.

Cirrhotic PVT

Occurs in up to 25% of patients due to a combination of decreased flow and an imbalance between anti-thrombotic and pro-thrombotic factors. Highest risk in patients with HCC. Can lead to hepatic decompensation (i.e. ascites, hepatic encephalopathy). Extension involving the mesenteric vessels is a poor prognostic sign.

Non-cirrhotic PVT

Can occur secondary to an underlying pro-thrombotic state, abdominal surgery, abdominal sepsis (more common in children), pancreatitis, tumour thrombus (classically from a renal cell carcinoma), infections (HIV), and drugs (azathioprine, didanosine).

Treatment

- Stop OCP.
- Varices should treated in the conventional manner: endoscopic management ± propranolol.
- Anticoagulation for a minimum of 3 months in patients with non-cirrhotic PVT. Start patient on low molecular weight heparin followed by oral anticoagulation when no invasive procedures are anticipated.
- Life-long anticoagulation in patients with an underlying pro-thrombotic defect.
- Anticoagulation in patients with cirrhosis can be beneficial but should be assessed on an individual case basis.
- Interval CT/MRI is required to assess for extension, dissolution or recanalisation.

Sinusoidal obstruction syndrome

Previously referred to as veno-occlusive disease. Occurs due to obstruction of the terminal hepatic venules and hepatic sinusoids. Injury begins in the centrilobular region of the liver lobule (zone 3). There is often associated fibrosis of sinusoidal walls. Most often occurs in patients undergoing haemopoietic cell transplantation (usually within 3 weeks; i.e. bone marrow, cord blood). Other scenarios include post-chemotherapy, use of certain medications (e.g. azathioprine, 6-mercaptopurine), ingestion of pyrrolizidine alkaloid toxins (bush tea), arsenic poisoning or post-liver transplantation. Clinical presentation is similar to Budd–Chiari syndrome. Circulatory obstruction usually precedes liver dysfunction.

Prophylaxis with low molecular weight heparin (prophylactic dosing) or UDCA (600–900 mg/day) is recommended. Treatment of established sinusoidal obstruction syndrome is difficult. TPA (recombinant tissue-type plasma plasminogen activator) and defibrotide have both been used. Defibrotide appears to be the most promising option. Severe sinusoidal obstruction syndrome is invariably fatal.

Ischaemic hepatitis

Also known as shock liver or hypoxic hepatitis. Occurs because of acute hypoperfusion and is a global hepatic injury. This condition is more common in patients with right-sided heart failure or in patients with COPD. Raised AST/ALT >1000 IU/mL is common. Usually self-limiting, although liver failure can occur and is more likely in patients with underlying liver disease. Treatment is supportive and aimed at restoring the systemic blood pressure and improving the haemodynamics.

Hepatic infarction

Occurs following a focal loss of blood supply resulting in focal ischaemic injury. Causes include embolic disease (e.g. endocarditis), thrombosis of the hepatic artery, iatrogenic ligation of the hepatic artery (e.g. at the time of laprascopic cholecystectomy), post radio-frequency ablation and following hepatic artery embolization (e.g. chemoembolization for HCC). A wedged-shaped infarct may be seen on CT/MRI. Treatment is usually supportive and directed towards the underlying cause.

Sickle cell hepatopathy

Acute manifestations include vaso-occlusive crises, sequestration crises and acute cholestasis due to hypoxic injury to hepatocytes. Concurrent sepsis is also common. Chronic manifestations include cholestasis, siderosis and cirrhosis. Liver biopsy is associated with an increased risk of bleeding. Liver transplantation may be an option.

40 Hepatocellular carcinoma

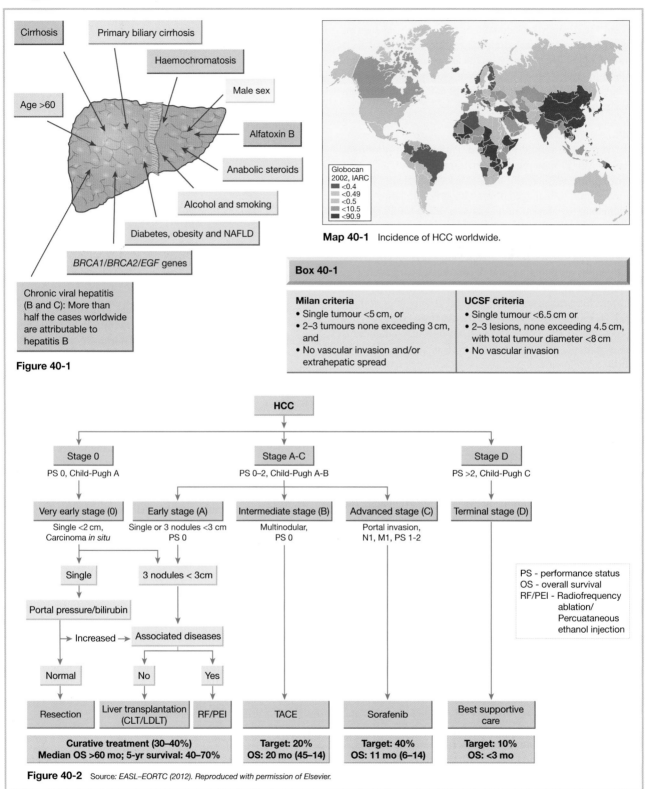

Cirrhosis

Primary biliary cirrhosis

Haemochromatosis

Male sex

Age >60

Alfatoxin B

Anabolic steroids

Alcohol and smoking

Diabetes, obesity and NAFLD

BRCA1/BRCA2/EGF genes

Chronic viral hepatitis (B and C): More than half the cases worldwide are attributable to hepatitis B

Figure 40-1

Globocan 2002, IARC
- <0.4
- <0.49
- <0.5
- <10.5
- <90.9

Map 40-1 Incidence of HCC worldwide.

Box 40-1

Milan criteria
- Single tumour <5 cm, or
- 2–3 tumours none exceeding 3 cm, and
- No vascular invasion and/or extrahepatic spread

UCSF criteria
- Single tumour <6.5 cm or
- 2–3 lesions, none exceeding 4.5 cm, with total tumour diameter <8 cm
- No vascular invasion

HCC

Stage 0
PS 0, Child-Pugh A

Stage A-C
PS 0–2, Child-Pugh A-B

Stage D
PS >2, Child-Pugh C

Very early stage (0)
Single <2 cm, Carcinoma *in situ*

Early stage (A)
Single or 3 nodules <3 cm
PS 0

Intermediate stage (B)
Multinodular, PS 0

Advanced stage (C)
Portal invasion, N1, M1, PS 1-2

Terminal stage (D)

Single

3 nodules < 3cm

Portal pressure/bilirubin

→ Increased →

Associated diseases

Normal

No

Yes

PS - performance status
OS - overall survival
RF/PEI - Radiofrequency ablation/ Percuataneous ethanol injection

Resection

Liver transplantation (CLT/LDLT)

RF/PEI

TACE

Sorafenib

Best supportive care

Curative treatment (30–40%)
Median OS >60 mo; 5-yr survival: 40–70%

Target: 20%
OS: 20 mo (45–14)

Target: 40%
OS: 11 mo (6–14)

Target: 10%
OS: <3 mo

Figure 40-2 Source: *EASL–EORTC (2012). Reproduced with permission of Elsevier.*

Hepatology at a Glance, First Edition. Deepak Joshi, Ceri Keane and Alison Brind.

Primary liver cancers

- 75–90% are hepatocellular carcinomas (HCC) and arise from the liver parenchyma.
- 10–25% are cholangiocarcinoma (CC) and arise from the epithelial lining of the bile ducts (see Chapter 41).
- Rare primary liver tumours include angiosarcomas and hepatoblastomas.

Hepatocellular carcinoma

Epidemiology

HCC is the sixth most common cancer worldwide, with an estimated 750 000 new cases per year. Incidence varies significantly between countries (see map). The highest prevalence is in China, South-East Asia, sub-Saharan and North Africa where carriage of chronic viral hepatitis is high. In Europe and North America, rates of chronic hepatitis and therefore HCC in the general population are comparatively lower. HCCs that arise from NASH and alcohol-related cirrhosis are becoming increasingly common in the West where prevalence of these diseases is steadily rising. Ninety per cent of HCCs are associated with one or more of the following risk factors:

- Age >60;
- Male sex;
- Chronic viral hepatitis (B and C): more than half the cases worldwide are attributable to hepatitis B;
- Cirrhosis;
- Haemochromatosis;
- Primary biliary cirrhosis;
- Alfatoxin B;
- Anabolic steroids;
- *BRCA1/BRCA2/EGF* genes;
- Alcohol and smoking; and
- Diabetes, obesity and NAFLD.

Clinical presentation

Patients with advanced liver cancer typically have symptoms of fatigue, weight loss, abdominal pain, pruritus, jaundice or decompensation. However, most patients with HCC are relatively asymptomatic until late in the disease.

Prevention of HCC

HCC surveillance, with a 6-monthly US is recommended in the following groups (EASL):

- Cirrhotic patients, Child–Pugh stage A or B;
- Cirrhotic patients, Child–Pugh stage C awaiting liver transplantation;
- Non-cirrhotic HBV carriers with active hepatitis or a family history of HCC;
- Non-cirrhotic patients with chronic hepatitis C and advanced liver fibrosis.

Investigations

Tumour markers: Alpha-fetoprotein (AFP): Although widely used, is only diagnostic of HCC when significantly elevated (>400 ng/mL). Not useful for surveillance as only 10–20% of small HCCs are associated with an abnormal AFP.

Abdominal ultrasound: A sensitivity of 58–89% for detecting HCC in high-risk groups. However, the test is operator-dependent and may miss small tumours.

Cross-sectional imaging: A staging CT of the chest, abdomen and pelvis is required in all malignant liver tumours to exclude metastatic disease. A contrast-enhanced CT or MRI is recommended if a nodule is found on surveillance US. HCC can be diagnosed without a biopsy in any nodules >2 cm that demonstrate 'venous washout'.

Liver biopsy: A liver biopsy is recommended for diagnosis in small liver nodules (1–2 cm) and liver lesions of any size that do not meet diagnostic radiological criteria for HCC. A liver biopsy is associated with a very small risk of tumour seeding or post-procedure bleeding.

Treatment

Treatment of primary liver tumours is dependent on:

- Tumour stage;
- Involvement of major vessels;
- The position of the lesion; and
- The patient's performance status and presence of cirrhosis.

To decide on the most appropriate treatment option for HCC, several staging criteria have been developed but the Barcelona Clinic Liver Cancer staging and treatment strategy is the most widely used (Figure 40.2).

Surgery: In patients with primary liver tumours and a normal liver or Child–Pugh A cirrhosis, resection is the first-line treatment. Perioperative mortality is 2–3% and 5-year survival can be up to 80% in well-selected patients.

Transplantation: Historically, liver transplantation for HCC has been associated with poor outcomes. The introduction of Milan criteria in 1996 (see Box 40.1) limited transplantation to small HCCs and was associated with a dramatic improvement in survival. The upper limit of tumour size when considering transplantation is controversial. Several extended criteria (e.g. University of California, San Francisco (UCSF) criteria), have been subsequently used without deterioration in overall survival.

Chemotherapy and radiotherapy: Systemic chemotherapy is rarely used in the treatment of HCC as less than one-fifth of tumours respond.

Biological therapies: (e.g. sorafenib, an oral multi-tyrosine kinase inhibitor) has been shown to improve survival in patients with advanced HCC. However, its use has currently not been approved by the National Institute for Clinical Excellence in the UK.

Local and ablative treatments: A range of local and ablative treatments for liver cancer have been developed (e.g. transarterial chemoembolisation and radiofrequency ablation). They are considered to be first-line therapies for patients with early or intermediate stage HCCs that are outside surgical criteria or in those who are unfit to undergo major surgery (Figure 40.2).

41 Cholangiocarcinoma

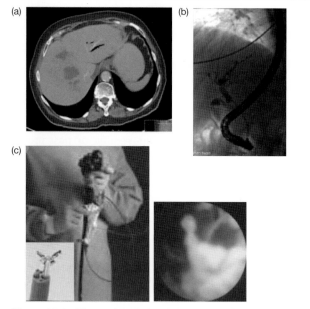

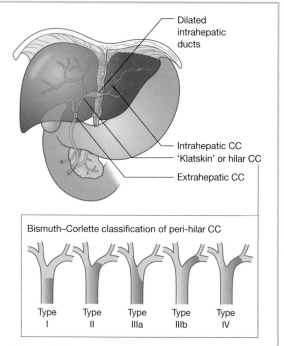

Figure 41-1 Diagnosing cholangiocarcinoma (CC).
(a) Cross-sectional imaging (e.g. CT and/or MRCP)
(b) ERCP + brushings
(c) Novel diagnostic tools (e.g. Spyglass cholangioscope system, Boston Scientific Corp, MA, USA) with cholangioscopic view of hilar CC. Source: *Keane MG, et al (2013).*

Figure 41-2

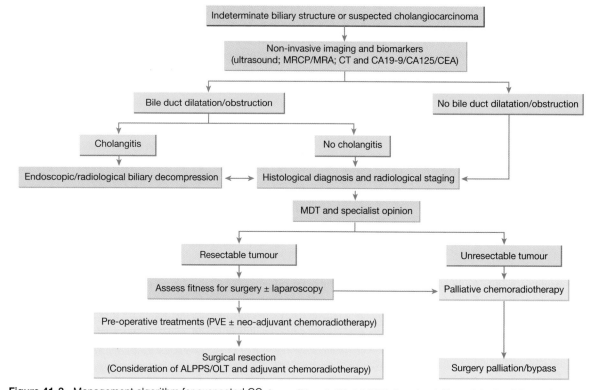

Figure 41-3 Management algorithm for suspected CC. Source: *Skipworth JRA et al. (2014). Reproduced with permission from S Karger AG, Basel.*

Epidemiology

Cholangiocarcinoma (CC) is a rare cancer arising from the lining of the gallbladder or bile ducts. Incidence of CC in the UK is approximately 1–2 per 100 000 population, but continues to increase annually (particularly rates of intrahepatic CC). In the mid-1990s CC overtook HCC as the leading cause of liver cancer death. Unlike HCC, most CC occur in a normal liver.

Established risk factors for CC

- Age >60;
- Male sex;
- Primary sclerosing cholangitis (PSC): 5–36% develop CC;
- Hepatolithiasis or choledocholitiasis;
- Bile duct adenoma or biliary papillomatosis;
- Congenital disorders (choledochal cysts or Caroli's disease);
- Parasitic infections (e.g. liver flukes such as *Opisthorchis viverrini* and *Clonorchis sinensis*). Worldwide, the highest prevalence of CC has been reported from northern Thailand and is attributed to these parasites;
- Cirrhosis;
- Chronic viral hepatitis (B and C);
- Toxins: dioxins, nitrosamines and vinyl chloride;
- Alcohol and smoking;
- Diabetes, obesity and NAFLD.

Presentation

CC can arise from the intrahepatic (5–10%), hilar (approximately 70%) or extrahepatic (20–30%) bile ducts. Hilar and extrahepatic tumours typically cause progressive biliary obstruction, leading to painless obstructive jaundice with or without cholangitis. Intrahepatic CCs form a solitary mass, which typically causes non-specific symptoms such as right upper quadrant pain, anorexia or nausea.

Classification

Hilar tumours can obstruct the right and left hepatic ducts and are classified according to the Bismuth–Corlette classification (Figure 41.2). CC is staged according to the tumour–node–metastasis system.

Investigations

Tumour markers, e.g. carbohydrate antigen 19-9 (CA19-9): CA19-9 is elevated in most patients with CC but is only suggestive of CC if persistently elevated after biliary decompression. (NB: approximately 7% of the population lack the necessary fucosyltransferase to produce CA19-9.)

Cross-sectional imaging: A staging CT of the chest, abdomen and pelvis determines local disease extent and distal spread. Contrast enhanced MRI/MRCP is complementary and used to further delineate biliary anatomy preoperatively or pre-stenting.

Histology: Cytological or histological confirmation can be obtained percutaneously or endoscopically via ERCP or EUS. However, standard brush cytology obtained by ERCP is only positive for malignancy in 9–57% of cases. Emerging cytological techniques such as fluorescence *in situ* hybridisation (FISH) and digital image analysis, which detect DNA abnormalities in brush cytology, are improving sensitivity. The diagnostic accuracy of biliary biopsies is also improving through the use of cholangioscopy (Figure 41.1).

Treatment

Surgery: Resection with clear pathological margins is associated with the best long-term survival in CC. Therefore an aggressive surgical approach with vascular reconstruction as necessary is the mainstay of treatment. However, less than one-third of patients have disease amenable to surgical resection at the time of diagnosis. In those suitable for surgery, preoperative biliary drainage is generally recommended in those with significant jaundice or cholangitis. Postoperatively, the most common cause of death in the short term is liver failure due a small liver remnant. To prevent this, increasingly portal vein embolisation or associating liver partition with portal vein ligation for staged hepatectomy (ALPPS) are used to promote hepatic hypertrophy of the future liver remnant (FLR) prior to resection. Type of liver resection is dependent on tumour site (see Chapter 42).

Transplantation: Liver transplantation is not routinely recommended for CC in the UK due to significant rates of recurrence. However, emerging evidence suggests that in combination with neoadjuvant chemotherapy outcomes may be comparable to HCC.

Chemotherapy and radiotherapy: In advanced CC not amenable to surgical resection, combination chemotherapy (cisplatin and gemcitabine) has been shown to improve overall survival. Following surgery, adjuvant chemotherapy is recommended for all patients with microscopically positive resection margins, as well as those with node-positive disease.

Palliative stenting: Biliary drainage is essential in CC to prevent cholangitis and enable patients to undergo palliative chemotherapy. Endoscopic or percutaneous biliary stenting is associated with shorter hospital stays and fewer complications than surgical decompression. Self-expanding metal stents (SEMS) have greater longevity than plastic stents. However, uncovered SEMS are permanent and often a plastic stent or removable covered metal stent is inserted while confirmation of malignancy is obtained.

Local and ablative treatments: Although well established in the management of HCC, these treatments have only occasionally been used in the treatment of CC, but early outcomes are promising.

Other rare primary liver cancers

Angiosarcoma: Arise from the cells lining the blood vessels of the liver. Treatment is by surgical resection in combination with chemotherapy.

Hepatoblastoma: Occur in children <4 years. If disease is limited to the liver patients often respond very well to a combination of surgery and chemotherapy.

42 Surgical procedures

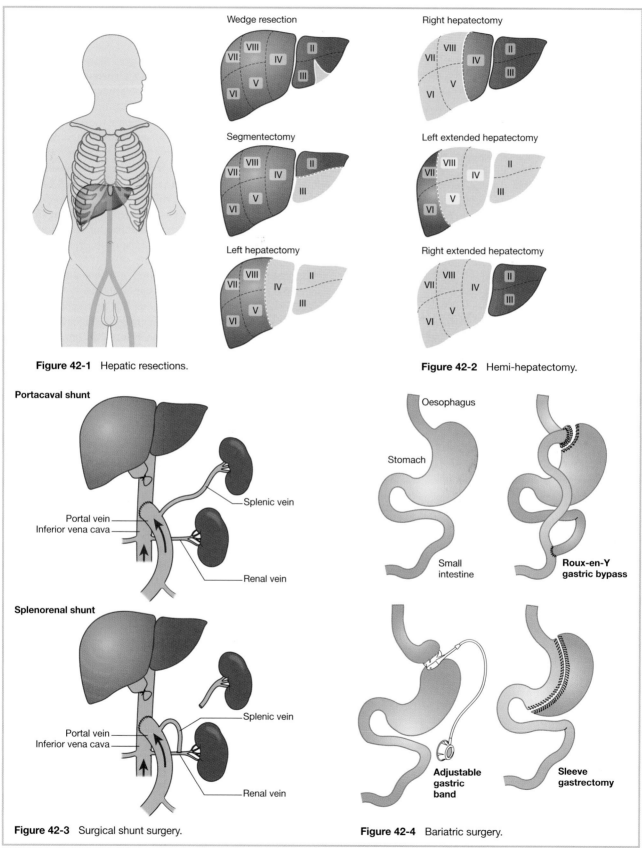

Figure 42-1 Hepatic resections.

Figure 42-2 Hemi-hepatectomy.

Figure 42-3 Surgical shunt surgery.

Figure 42-4 Bariatric surgery.

Hepatology at a Glance, First Edition. Deepak Joshi, Geri Keane and Alison Brind.
© 2015 John Wiley & Sons, Ltd. Published 2015 by John Wiley & Sons, Ltd. Companion website: www.ataglanceseries.com/hepatology

The role of the hepato-biliary surgeon is integral to the multidisciplinary team approach to patients with CLD and its complications. However, surgery in patients with liver disease is associated with an increased frequency of surgical and anaesthetic complications compared to patients without liver disease. Patients with a Child–Pugh score >8 or a MELD score >10 are more likely to develop complications as are Child–Pugh class A patients with portal hypertension. Abdominal surgery carries the greatest risk. Surgery should be performed in experienced centres.

Surgical aspects of liver transplantation have been described in Chapter 22. Understanding the segmental and vascular supply is important to how surgery can be performed. Major liver surgery is usually performed through a 'roof-top' incision to allow optimal access and exposure to the liver and major blood vessels. Some surgery can be performed laparascopically.

Hepatic resection

Resections of the liver can be performed for benign or malignant lesions but most are performed for primary or secondary tumours. Improved surgical techniques and improved perioperative and postoperative care has led to improved outcomes. Most surgery begins laparoscopically to assess whether resection is possible before performing bilateral sub-costal incisions. Intraoperative US is also performed to examine the liver to ensure the patient's disease has not progressed.

Wedge resection

A non-anatomical resection usually performed for small lesions at the periphery of the liver open ot laparoscopically. A V-shaped portion is removed.

Segmental resection

An anatomical resection of one or more segments of the liver. Removal of multiple segments is referred to as sectorectomy.

Hemi-hepatectomy

A left or right hemi-hepatectomy can be performed. An extended left hepatectomy involves removal of the left lobe (segments II, III and IV) and segments V and VIII. An extended right hepatectomy involves removal of the right lobe (segments V, VI, VII and VIII) and the caudate lobe (segment I) and segment IV. Extended hepatectomies are technically challenging and a reasonable volume liver remnant is required in order for the patient to recover. If an insufficient volume of liver remains then the patient can develop a functional 'small for size' syndrome (hyperbilirubinaemia, coagulopathy and hepatic encephalopathy). Essentially, the residual functional liver volume is too small for the patient and is unable to perform the normal liver functions.

An alternative to portal vein embolisation is associating liver partition with portal vein ligation for staged hepatectomy (ALPPS). This achieves more rapid growth of the FLR, enabling resection of tumours that would have been previously been considered unresectable. This two-stage technique involves initial *in situ* transection of liver parenchyma (along the intended line of hepatic resection) with portal vein ligation, followed by completion hepatectomy 7–14 days later.

Surgical shunts

Portacaval shunt

Involves the anastomosis of the portal vein to the inferior vena cava. Usually performed for uncontrollable variceal bleeding resulting in a decrease in portal pressure. Not performed commonly mainly due to the improved outcomes with TIPS.

Splenorenal shunt

Involves a splenectomy followed by anastomosis of the splenic vein to the left renal vein. Indications include portal hypertension and uncontrollable bleeding from oesophageal and gastric varices. Uncommon procedure.

LeVeen peritoneovenous shunt

Used for the management of diuretic resistant ascites although not performed commonly. Involves the surgical implantation of a perforated catheter in the peritoneal cavity which is then connected to the superior vena cava/jugular vein. A one-way valve is also inserted subcutaneously which controls the direction of ascites and prevents a back-flow of blood.

Bariatric surgery

The increasing obesity epidemic has led to the development of surgical techniques to help achieve sustained weight loss. Weight loss is achieved by either malabsorption or restriction or both.

Roux-en-Y gastric bypass

Can be performed laparoscopically. Weight loss is achieved by a combination of restriction and malabsorption. Most commonly performed weight loss surgery. Also results in decrease production of ghrelin (appetite-stimulating peptide hormone), and increased production of appetite-suppressing glucagon-like peptide-1 (GLP-1).

Sleeve gastrectomy

Involves removal of the greater curve of the stomach and creation of a tubular stomach. Weight loss is achieved by restriction. Ghrelin levels also decrease and GLP-1 levels increase.

Adjustable gastric band

Involves the placement of a tight adjustable prosthetic band around the fundus of the stomach. A locking silicone ring is also placed in the subcutaneous tissue which allows the band diameter to be adjusted following the injection of saline. Weight loss is achieved through restriction.

43 Biliary disorders

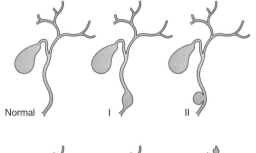

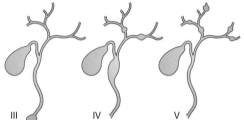

Normal   I   II

III   IV   V

Figure 43-1   Classification of choledochal cysts.
I, common type; II, diverticulum; III, choledochocoele;
IV, multiple cysts (intra- and extrahepatic); V, intrahepatic
duct cysts (Caroli's disease).

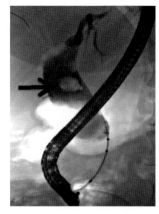
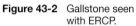

Figure 43-2   Gallstone seen
with ERCP.

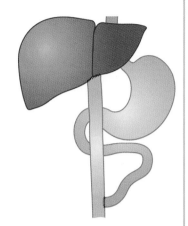

Figure 43-4   Kasai procedure.

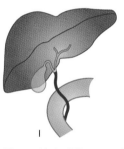
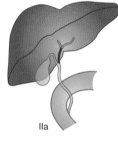
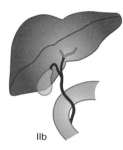
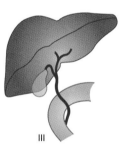

I   IIa   IIb   III

Figure 43-3   Biliary atresia.

Hepatology at a Glance, First Edition. Deepak Joshi, Geri Keane and Alison Brind.

Biliary disorders
Gallstones

Gallstones occur in approximately 10% of men and women but largely remain asymptomatic. Gallstones that remain in the gallbladder may cause biliary colic (constant right upper quadrant pain). Triggers include a fatty meal which causes gallbladder contractions. Gallstones appear as echogenic foci and cast an acoustic shadow on abdominal US. Sludge and gravel can also be seen on US. Patients with typical symptoms of biliary pain who have a normal US should have either an EUS or MRCP.

Common complications of gallstone disease include acute cholecystitis, choledocholithiasis, cholangitis, biliary obstruction and pancreatitis. Rarer complications include gallstone ileus, Bouveret's syndrome (gastric outlet obstruction secondary to an impacted gallstone in pylorus or proximal duodenum) and Mirizzi's syndrome (impacted gallstone in the cystic duct leading to biliary obstruction).

Acute cholecystitis

The most common complication. Patients present with right upper quadrant (RUQ) pain and fever. Murphy's sign (RUQ discomfort/pain on inspiration) is positive. Abdominal US findings include gallbladder wall thickening or oedema. Treatment is with antibiotics initially and then cholecystectomy.

Choledocholithiasis

Refers to patients with stones within the common bile duct or the intrahepatic biliary tree. Patients usually present with pain. If biliary obstruction occurs then patients develop jaundice and raised ALP/GGT which can then lead to acute cholangitis (raised WCC, fever, sepsis). An abdominal US scan is recommended first line which can demonstrate dilatation of the common bile duct (>10 mm in patients who have had a cholecystectomy; otherwise >7 mm). An MRCP or EUS may be required to confirm the diagnosis. An ERCP will be required in patients with confirmed stones.

Caroli's disease

A congenital disorder (autosomal recessive) characterised by multifocal segmental dilatation of the intrahepatic biliary tree. It is regarded as a type of choledochal cyst (type V). It is commonly associated with renal cysts, in particular autosomal recessive adult polycystic kidney disease. Two variants are described: Caroli's disease and Caroli's syndrome. Caroli's disease is less common and is characterised by bile duct ectasia without other liver parenchymal abnormalities. Caroli's syndrome is more common and is associated with congenital hepatic fibrosis. Dilatation of the biliary tree predisposed patients to biliary sludge, intraductal stone formation and recurrent cholangitis. Secondary biliary cirrhosis can also occur. Diagnosis is based on imaging (US, CT or MRI) which demonstrates bile duct ectasia and irregular cystic dilatation of the large proximal intrahepatic bile ducts but with a normal common bile duct. Management is supportive. Courses of rotating antibiotics for recurrent cholangitis may be required. Patients with end-stage liver disease and its complications may require consideration for liver transplantation. Prognosis is variable and is dependent on the degree of liver synthetic dysfunction and renal dysfunction.

Biliary atresia

Biliary atresia (BAT) is a rare idiopathic disorder affecting neonates only. It is characterised by a destructive inflammatory obliterative cholangiopathy affecting both the intrahepatic and extrahepatic ducts. It is more common in patients from East Asia. Untreated, liver cirrhosis occurs leading to death by the age of 2 years. It is the most common indication for liver transplantation in children. BAT can be divided into three categories:
- *BAT without anomalies or malformations*: also known as perinatal BAT. Accounts for 85% of cases. Jaundice occurs within first 2 months of life.
- *BAT with laterality malformations*: also known as biliary atresia splenic malformation. Occurs in 10–15% of BAT cases. Laterality malformations include situs inversus, asplenia, absence of the inferior vena cava and intestinal malformation.
- *BAT in combination with congenital malformations*: occurs in 5–10% of BAT cases and is associated with intestinal atresia, kidney abnormalities and heart malformations.

Most children are born at full term with a normal birth weight. Jaundice develops usually by the eighth week with pale stools and dark urine. Blood tests demonstrate a conjugated hyperbilirubinaemia, raised aminotransferases, a disproportionately increased GGT and a raised INR (usually due to concurrent vitamin K deficiency). US is required to exclude other causes of cholestasis and identify other features associated with BAT – abnormal size and shape of gallbladder, absence of the common bile duct and the 'triangular cord' sign (triangular echogenic density seen above the porta hepatitis). A liver biopsy may be helpful in excluding histological changes consistent with other causes of intrahepatic cholestasis. The diagnosis of BAT is made by a cholangiogram – ERCP or surgical cholangiogram. If BAT is confirmed then a Kasai procedure is required (hepatoportoenterostomy). Jaundice should improve within weeks. If jaundice remains 3 months after surgery then the patient should be referred for liver transplant assessment. Post-Kasai, patients will require UDCA and fat-soluble vitamin supplementation. Complications include cholangitis and portal hypertension due to progressive biliary cirrhosis. Most patients with BAT will eventually require liver transplantation.

Sphincter of Oddi dysfunction

Sphincter of Oddi dysfunction (SOD) is a benign condition which results from acalculous obstruction to biliary/pancreatic outflow through the sphincter of Oddi. SOD encompasses both sphincter of Oddi stenosis and dyskinesia and is also a cause of recurrent pancreatitis. It occurs in approximately 1% of the general population. Classification is according to the Milwaukee classification (types I–III). Imaging can help exclude other causes (i.e. gallstones). Sphincter of Oddi manometry remains the gold standard to diagnose SOD – elevated biliary and pancreatic pressures >40 mmHg. Patients with elevated pressures require sphincterotomy (biliary or pancreatic respectively). Improvement in patient symptoms is variable. SOM is associated with an increased risk of pancreatitis and should be performed in specialist centres only.

44 Pancreatic disorders

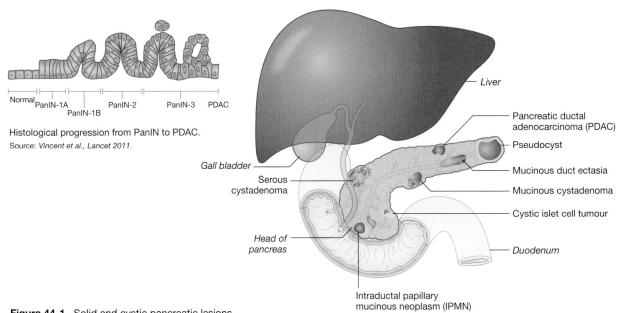

Histological progression from PanIN to PDAC.

Source: *Vincent et al., Lancet 2011.*

Figure 44-1 Solid and cystic pancreatic lesions.

Table 44-1 Characteristics of pancreatic lesions.

	PDAC	IPMN	MCN	SCA	Pseudocyst
Age	Elderly	Elderly	Middle age	Middle age/elderly	Any
Gender	>50% male	70% male	95% female	>50% female	>50% male
Common presenting symptoms	Pain Jaundice Weight loss	Asymptomatic Pain Jaundice	Asymptomatic Pain	Asymptomatic Pain (associated with von Hippel–Lindau syndrome)	Pain, nausea + vomiting post episode of acute pancreatitis
Location in pancreas	Anywhere	Head (70%), can be multifocal	Body/tail (95%)	Anywhere	Anywhere
Lesion	Irregular solid mass	Cyst	Cyst	Cyst + central stellate scar	Cyst
Communication with pancreatic duct	Sometimes	Common	No	No	Common

Hepatology at a Glance, First Edition. Deepak Joshi, Geri Keane and Alison Brind.

Pancreatic cancer

Epidemiology

Pancreatic ductal adenocarcinoma (PDAC) is the 10th most common cancer but the fifth most common cause of cancer death in the UK. PDAC is invariably diagnosed late and at an advanced stage when curative surgical resection is no longer possible. Risk factors for PDAC include smoking, family history, chronic pancreatitis, diabetes and obesity.

Pathogenesis

Pancreatic cancers may arise from the exocrine or endocrine portions of the gland. Most tumours (>90%) arise from the exocrine cells (e.g. the ductal epithelium, acinar cells, connective tissue and lymphatic tissue). PDAC develops as a consequence of the progressive accumulation of somatic genetic mutations (e.g. KRAS2, CDKN2, p53 or SMAD4). Progressive histological changes seen within the ductal epithelium reflect the accumulation of somatic mutations; normal ductal epithelium advances through a series of dysplastic stages to develop ultimately into adenocarcinoma (Figure 44.1).

Diagnosis

Symptoms: Three-quarters of tumours arise in the head of the pancreas. As the tumour grows, it often leads to occlusion of the common bile duct and infiltration or obstruction of the duodenum. Patients develop jaundice, weight loss, anorexia, abdominal and/or back pain. Many symptoms overlap with a variety of other conditions and diagnosing PDAC in the early stages remains a challenge.

Investigations: Unlike other cancers there are no simple screening tests for PDAC. Patients may develop abnormal liver biochemistry, an elevated glucose or rising tumour markers (e.g. CA19-9). The imaging modality of choice is CT (pancreas protocol) or MRI as US views of the pancreas are often obscured. Screening and surveillance by EUS may have a role in high-risk individuals (e.g. strong family history of PDAC, hereditary pancreatitis or those with Peutz–Jeghers syndrome or p16, BRAC2 and hereditary non-polyposis colorectal cancer mutation carriers), who are at an increased risk of developing PDAC.

Treatment

Surgical resection with adjuvant chemotherapy is the only curative therapy for PDAC. However, only 10–20% of patients have disease that is amenable to surgery at the time of diagnosis and most patients are managed by palliative biliary stenting, chemotherapy and/or radiotherapy. Pancreatic exocrine insufficiency is also common and often under-treated with enzyme supplementation.

Prognosis

Overall 5-year survival is <4%. Those diagnosed with disease amenable to surgical resection have improved survival but recurrence is common and fewer than one-third will survive 5 years.

Pancreatic cystic tumours

Pancreatic cysts are an increasingly common finding, found in 1.2–2.6% of patients undergoing CT and up to 13.5% undergoing MRI for non-pancreatic indications. They have a wide differential diagnosis, including inflammatory cysts such as pseudocysts, benign cysts such as serocyst adenomas (SCA) and premalignant cysts such as intraductal papillary mucinous neoplasms (IPMN) and mucinous cystadenomas (MCN). Pancreatic cysts are often asymptomatic but may obstruct the pancreatic duct leading to pain and pancreatitis, or the common bile duct leading to jaundice.

Cross-sectional imaging±EUS-FNA are used to differentiate benign and premalignant cystic lesions of the pancreas.

Pseudocysts complicate 16–50% cases of acute pancreatitis but typically resolve over time. If they remain symptomatic, pseudocysts can be drained percutaneously, endoscopically (EUS-guided cystgastrostomy) or surgically.

Approximately 8% of cases of PDAC arise from premalignant cystic tumours of the pancreas (i.e. IPMN and MCN). Regular surveillance of these and any indeterminate cystic lesions is therefore recommended in accordance with international guidance.

Pancreatic neuroendocrine tumours

Pancreatic neuroendocrine tumours (PNETs) are rare tumours that arise from the pancreatic islet cells. Two-thirds of PNETs are functional and secrete hormones (e.g. gastrin, insulin, glucagon, vasoactive intestinal polypeptide and somotostatin), and present with a clinical syndrome associated with excess hormone release. PNETs are often associated with recognised clinical syndromes such as multiple endocrine neoplasia, von Hippel–Lindau syndrome, neurofibromatosis type 1 and tuberous sclerosis. Typically, PNETs are managed by surgical resection±somatostatin analogues and chemotherapy.

Acute pancreatitis

Acute pancreatitis (AP) has an incidence of 5–25 per 100 000 population. Causes of AP include:

- Gallstones;
- Alcohol;
- Hypertriglyceridaemia;
- Hypercalcaemia;
- Hereditary pancreatitis;
- Post-ERCP;
- Infectious (e.g. mumps, coxsackie virus);
- Pancreatic duct obstruction (e.g. ampullary stenosis, PDAC, SOD and parasites, e.g. ascaris);
- Scorpion bites;
- Autoimmune pancreatitis; and
- Idiopathic.

Management

Clinical scoring systems (e.g. Ranson or Glasgow criteria) are used to assess the severity of pancreatitis. Approximately 20–30% of cases of AP are classified as severe, characterised by the presence of pancreatic necrosis. In severe AP, mortality is 30–40% compared to 1% in mild AP. Patients with severe AP should therefore be managed in a HDU/ITU setting with joint medical and surgical input to advise on best supportive care, drainage of collections and/or timing of necrosectomy as necessary.

Chronic pancreatitis

Chronic pancreatitis is characterised by chronic inflammation, calcification and atrophy of the pancreas. It is caused by alcohol in >75% of cases. The early disease is dominated by chronic abdominal pain, with time pain diminishes and exocrine and endocrine insufficiency dominate.

Complications

- Portal vein thrombosis with portal hypertension;
- Low biliary stricture causing jaundice;
- Pancreatic pseudocyst;
- Gastric outlet obstruction;
- Pancreatic cancer (eightfold increased risk).

45 Post-liver transplantation: general considerations

Table 45-1

Agent	Class of drug	Mechanism of action	Common side effects
Prednisolone	Glucocorticosteroid	Suppressed T-cell activity, macrophages and leucocytes	↑ BP, hyperlipidaemia, ↑ glucose osteoporosis, mood swings, peptic ulceration
Tacrolimus	Calcineurin inhibitor	↓ IL-2, inhibits T-cell activation	↑ BP, insulin resistance, renal dysfunction, hyperlipidaemia, neuropathy, tremor
Ciclosporin	Calcineurin inhibitor	↓ IL-2, inhibits T-cell activation	↑ BP, insulin resistance, renal dysfunction, hyperlipidaemia, neuropathy, tremor, gingival hyperplasia, hirsuitism
Azathioprine	Purine analogue	Inhibits adenosine and guanine production, inhibits DNA and RNA synthesis in proliferating T cells	Pancytopenia, pancreatitis, nausea, hepatitis
Mycophenolate mofetil	IMPDH inhibitor	Inhibits T and B cell proliferation	Gastrointestinal side effcts, rash, leucopenia, anaemia
Sirolimus/ Everolimus	mTOR inhibitor	Inhibits T-cell replication	Hyperlipidaemia, poor wound healing, hepatic artery thrombosus, leucopenia, vasculitis
Basiliximab	IL-2 inhibitor	IL-2 receptor blockade	Infections, pulmonary oedema

Table 45-2

Complication	Timing post transplant
Biliary leak	0–3 months
Anastomotic stricture	1–12 months
Non anastomic stricture	1–6 months
Biliary stones, sludge, casts	> 12 months

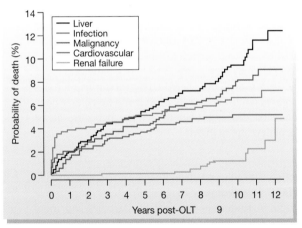

Figure 45-1 Primary cause of death over time post liver transplant.
Source: *Watt KDS et al. (2010).*
Reproduced with permission of John Wlley & Sons Ltd.

Hepatology at a Glance, First Edition. Deepak Joshi, Geri Keane and Alison Brind.
© 2015 John Wiley & Sons, Ltd. Published 2015 by John Wiley & Sons, Ltd. Companion website: www.ataglanceseries.com/hepatology

Immunosuppression

Choice of immunosuppression depends on a variety of factors including:

- Comorbidities;
- Previous experience/side-effects with immunosuppression;
- Indication for LT (e.g. sirolimus is advocated for patients with HCC);
- Likelihood of pregnancy (mycophenolate mofetil and sirolimus are teratogenic).

Combination immunosuppression, a calcineurin inhibitor (CNI, i.e. tacrolimus or ciclosporin) and steroids (prednisone) are usually used first-line. Monitoring of trough levels of CNIs are required to ensure adequate dosing and reduce toxicity. Target levels after 3 months are 5–10 ng/mL for tacrolimus and 100–150 ng/mL for ciclosporin. Other immunosuppressants (azathioprine, mycophenalate mofetil) may be added later. Other agents such as evorolimus, sirolimus (mTOR inhibitors) and interleukin-2 blockers (e.g. basiliximab) can also be used. Mode of action and common side effects of immunosuppression are listed in Table 45.1. Drug–drug interactions are common with immunosuppressive agents. Doses of immunosuppressive drugs need to be balanced and weighed against graft function, side effects and renal function, especially with CNIs. Immunosuppression is invariably lifelong; in rare instances patients develop immune tolerance to graft.

Cellular rejection

Can be divided into hyperacute (rare but due to preformed antibodies, e.g. ABO incompatibility), acute (occurs in approximately one-third of patients within the first 3 months) and chronic (progressive loss of bile ducts or ductopenia leading to graft failure). Acute cellular rejection (ACR) can be asymptomatic or present with pyrexia and RUQ pain. Liver biochemistry is abnormal (rising AST/ALT, bilirubin, ALP). A liver biopsy is required to confirm ACR and chronic rejection. ACR is characterised by the triad of endothelititis, bile duct damage and a lymphocytic portal inflammatory infiltrate. Treatment of ACR is with augmentation of immunosuppression ± use of high dose intravenous steroid depending on the severity.

General advice

Simple measures can help patients post-LT: regular exercise, smoking cessation, avoiding unnecessary sun exposure and frequent hand-washing. Pregnancy is possible but female LT recipients of childbearing age should undergo counselling regarding contraception.

Complications
Early (<3 months)

Primary non-function (acidosis, rising INR, transaminases and creatinine) occurs when the new liver fails to function normal. Primary non-function in the absence of hepatic artery thrombosis (HAT) is an indication of emergency retransplantation. HAT can lead to biliary leaks, hepatic necrosis and sepsis and is more common in paediatric patients due to the use of smaller vessels. Biliary complications are common as the hepatic artery exclusively provides the blood supply of the biliary tree. Doppler US is a sensitive screening tool.

Infections

The greatest number deaths occur soon after LT with nearly two-thirds of deaths are attributed to infection, intra-, peri- or postoperative. Highest risk is immediately post-LT (bacterial, fungal and protozoal) but can occur at any time point. CMV viraemia is common although end-organ disease is rare. Prophylactic antivirals (valganciclovir) are often given for 3 months in high-risk patients (i.e. donor positive, recipient negative). Patients should undergo vaccination pre-transplant and require annual influenza and pneumococcal vaccinations. Live vaccines should be avoided.

Biliary complications

Biliary complications are common post-LT. Often referred to as the 'Achilles heel' of LT. Timings of possible biliary complications are listed in Table 45.2.

Long-term (>12 months)
Cardiovascular disease and metabolic syndrome

There is an increased incidence of cardiovascular disease post-LT and is potentiated by the use of steroids and CNIs. Arterial hypertension (>140/90 mmHg; target BP 130/80 mmHg), hyperlipidaemia and insulin resistance/diabetes are common and should be treated aggressively. Cardiovascular disease is a common cause of death long-term post-LT.

Renal dysfunction

Acute and chronic renal dysfunction is common. The incidence of chronic kidney disease at 3 years is 14% and 18% at 5 years. Causes are multifactorial but include hypertension, diabetes mellitus and CNI toxicity. CNI-induced acute renal dysfunction occurs due to renal vasoconstriction and should improve with dose reduction. CNI-induced chronic renal dysfunction does not improve following dose reduction. Substituting the CNI for another agent (e.g. mycophenolate mofetil or sirolimus) may result in an improvement in renal function. Patients receiving CNIs should avoid NSAIDs, and due care should be taken with aminoglycosides.

Malignancy

Malignancy is a common cause of mortality long-term post-LT. Malignant tumours especially skin malignancies are frequent. Post-transplant lymphoproliferative disorder although rare can also occur (specific B-cell lymphoma). Patients transplanted for ALD are at increased risk of developing oropharygeal and oesophageal squamous cell carcinomas. Patients require colonoscopy 3 years after LT and then every 3–5 years.

Diabetes

New onset diabetes mellitus (NODM) is common post-SOT affecting 3–25% of patients. Risk factors for NODM include age >50 years, BMI >25, HCV infection, increased donor age and use of tacrolimus and steroids. Management of NODM should be as patients with type 2 diabetes.

46 Post-liver transplantation: disease recurrence

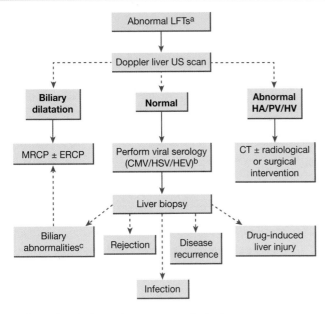

Table 46-1

Disease	Recurrence?	Graft loss?
AIH	✓	✓
HBV	✗	✗
HCV	✓	✓
NASH	✓	✗
PBC	✓	✗
PSC	✓	✓

[a] In setting of adequate immunosuppression levels
[b] HBV/HCV serology in patients transplanted for these aetiologies
[c] Ensure patency of hepatic artery

Figure 46-1 Investigation and management of abnormal LFTs post-liver transplant.

Hepatology at a Glance, First Edition. Deepak Joshi, Geri Keane and Alison Brind.

Abnormal liver function tests

A very common occurrence. An investigational algorithm is provided in Figure 46.1.

Recurrent disease

Certain disease cannot recur as the underlying metabolic defect has been removed (i.e. Wilson's disease). ALD may recur. HCC can recur as well develop *de novo* in grafts with recurrent cirrhosis.

Autoimmune hepatitis

Recurs in 20–30% of patients. *De novo* autoimmune hepatitis (AIH) has also been described post-LT particularly in patients undergoing HCV treatment with PEG-IFN. Recurrent AIH is diagnosed using autoantibody titres (>1 : 40) and liver biopsy. Treatment involves augmenting immunosuppression. Outcomes are good post-LT. A protocol liver biopsy is recommended at 5-year intervals. Retransplantation may be required.

Alcohol-related liver disease

Patients transplanted for alcohol can relapse and return to drinking. Risk factors for recidivism include no social support and length of abstinence pre-transplant. However, the majority of patients remain abstinent. Patients who return to levels of harmful drinking are at risk of alcoholic hepatitis, cirrhosis and pancreatitis and reduced survival rates are due to liver-related causes. Patients transplanted for alcohol and HCV have poorer survival rates than patients transplanted for alcohol alone. Patients who relapse need to engage with alcohol liaison services.

Hepatitis B virus

HBV-related cirrhosis has become an uncommon indication for LT in the Western world given the use of highly efficacious oral antiviral therapy (AVT). However, HCC on a background of HBV as an indication for LT has become more frequent. Survival post-LT is excellent; 10-year graft and patient survival of nearly 80%. This excellent survival rate is due to the combination use of hepatitis B immunoglobulin (HBIG) and oral nucleos(t)ide analogues. Low risk patients (i.e. undetectable HBV viral load at time of LT, good adherence, HBeAg negative at time of LT) can discontinue their HBIG post-LT and continue on oral AVT alone. Recurrence of HBV can occur post-LT and is usually due to failure of prophylactic therapy. The most severe form of recurrence, although very uncommon currently, is a fibrosing cholestatic recurrence of HBV which is characterised by high intrahepatic HBV titres, hepatocyte ballooning and cholestasis.

Hepatitis C virus

HCV recurrence is universal post-LT in patients with a detectable HCV viral load at the time of transplantation. Reinfection occurs at the time of retransplantation. Most patients develop a hepatitis within 3 months of transplant. Recurrent HCV is associated with inferior patient and graft survival post-LT than patients transplanted for other aetiologies. Risk factors for recurrence and a rapid recurrence of HCV include ACR requiring steroid boluses, diabetes, older donors, CMV infection and HIV co-infection. Fibrosis rates are accelerated post-LT resulting in recurrent cirrhosis in 30% of patients within 5–10 years. .

A protocol of 12-monthly liver biopsy is recommended. Indications for treatment of HCV post-LT include a cholestatic recurrence of HCV (usually occurs with 6–12 weeks post-LT) and evidence of progressive disease (≥F2). AVT with PEG-IFN and ribavirin is associated with inferior SVR rates and increased side effects including ACR. Dose reductions of tacrolimus and ciclosporin are required when using boceprevir and telaprevir. The newer DAAs have only been used in clinical trials but will undoubtedly improve SVR rates with a more favourable side-effect profile. Retransplantation may be an option for patients with recurrent cirrhosis.

NAFLD

Both NASH and NAFLD can reoccur or develop *de novo*. *De novo* disease is due to immunosuppression, all of which promote the metabolic syndrome. Risk factors for NAFLD include features of the metabolic syndrome pre-LT and steatosis on the allograft sample. Recurrent disease presents with abnormal liver biochemistry. A liver biopsy is required to diagnose recurrence and determine fibrosis grade. Treatment is by modification of risk factors for the metabolic syndrome (i.e. weight loss, exercise, treating hypertension, diabetes and hyperlipidaemia).

Primary biliary cirrhosis

Outcomes post-LT for PBC are excellent with some of the best reported graft and patient survival rates in the post-LT period. Positive AMA and raised IgM can persist post-transplant. Recurrent PBC affects approximately 20% of patients at median time of 3 years.

The diagnosis is made on liver biopsy. The use of ciclosporin has been associated with less severe disease recurrence than with tacrolimus. Although recurrent PBC may lead to abnormal liver biochemistry and graft dysfunction it does not have a negative impact on patient or graft survival. UDCA can improve liver biochemistry but does not improve patient or graft survival. Retransplantation is rarely required.

Primary sclerosing cholangitis

Good long-term outcomes are reported with PSC post-LT. All patients with PSC will have a Roux-en-Y biliary anastomosis to remove the risk of cholangiocarcinoma from the native bile duct. Recurrence of PSC in 50% of patients by 5 years. Risk factors for recurrent PSC include male sex, CMV infection, an intact colon and/or active IBD at the time of transplantation and steroid-resistant rejection. The diagnosis of recurrent PSC is made by using the combination of cholestatic liver enzymes, histology and characteristic cholangiography in the absence of other causes (i.e. infection, HAT). No treatments are available to attenuate the progression of disease. Patients with IBD require annual colonoscopy due to the high risk of developing colonic polyps and cancer. One-third of patients will require retransplantation.

47 Tropical liver disease: parenchymal

Countries or areas at high risk
Countries or areas at low risk

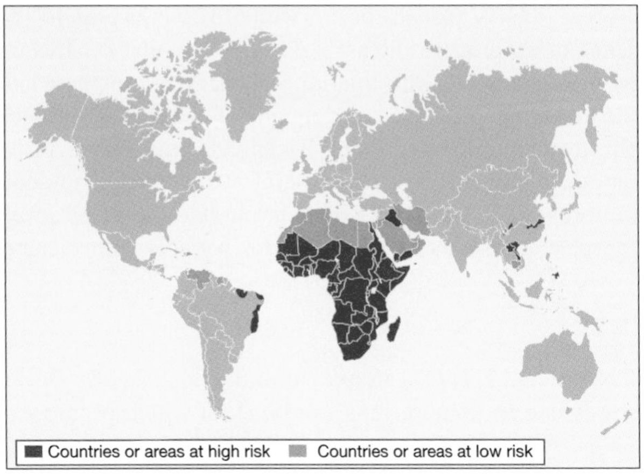

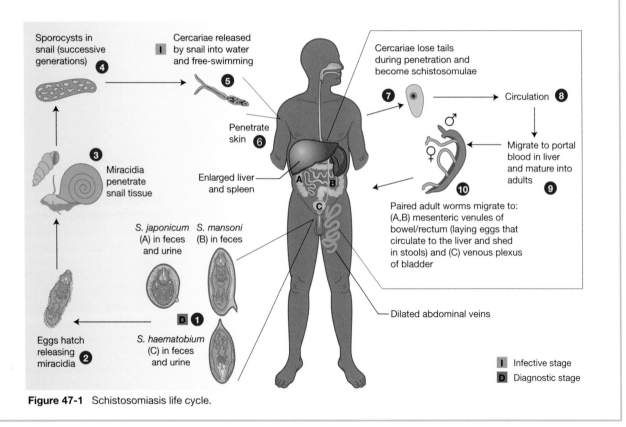

Map 47-1 Schistosomiasis.
Countries or areas at risk, 2007. *Source: Reproduced with permission of WHO.*

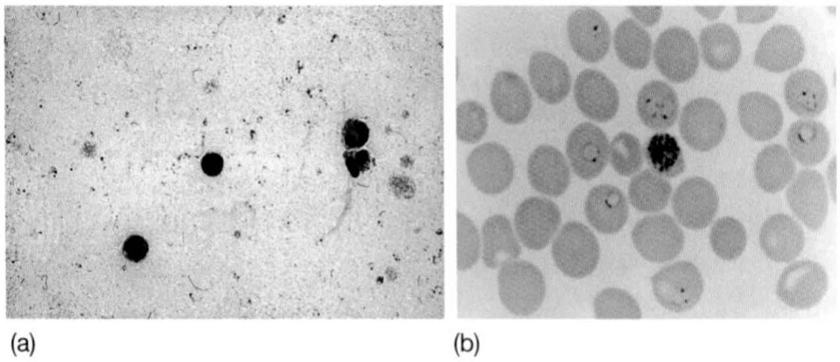

(a)
(b)

Figure 47-2 Malaria.
Thick and thin blood films in *Plasmodium falciparum*:
(a) thick film shows trophozoites + schizont;
(b) thin film shows ring trophozoites.
Source: *Beeching N & Gill G (2014). Reproduced with permission of John Wiley & Sons Ltd.*

Sporocysts in snail (successive generations) 4
I Cercariae released by snail into water and free-swimming
5
Penetrate skin 6
3
Miracidia penetrate snail tissue
Enlarged liver and spleen
A
B
C
S. japonicum (A) in feces and urine
S. mansoni (B) in feces
D 1
Eggs hatch releasing miracidia 2
S. haematobium (C) in feces and urine
Cercariae lose tails during penetration and become schistosomulae
7
Circulation 8
♂
♀
Migrate to portal blood in liver and mature into adults 9
10
Paired adult worms migrate to: (A,B) mesenteric venules of bowel/rectum (laying eggs that circulate to the liver and shed in stools) and (C) venous plexus of bladder
Dilated abdominal veins
I Infective stage
D Diagnostic stage

Figure 47-1 Schistosomiasis life cycle.

A variety of additional causes of jaundice and liver disease are found in patients living within the tropics or returning from overseas. Clinical history and geographical setting are essential when determining aetiology.

Abnormal LFTs and/or jaundice

Malaria

Jaundice, due to haemolysis, is a common feature. Blood film examination is diagnostic (Figure 47.2). For management see: UK malaria treatment guidelines in further reading.

Typhoid and paratyphoid enteric fevers

Typhoid is the second most common serious tropical disease seen in returning travelers, after malaria. It occurs following infection with *Salmonella* (*S. typhi* – typhoid; *S. paratyphi* types ABC – paratyphoid), which are highly prevalent in India and South-East Asia, sub-Saharan Africa, Central and South America. Patients present with fever, headache, cough, diarrhoea or constipation. LFTs are often abnormal. Blood cultures are usually diagnostic. Early antibiotic treatment with IV ceftriaxone or oral azithromycin is recommended to prevent complications (e.g. encephalopathy and gastrointestinal bleeding).

Viral hepatitis

See Chapters 28–30.

Human immunodeficiency virus

Patients with HIV are susceptible to hepatitis co-infection, invasive non-tuberculous mycobacterial or, rarely, cryptococcal hepatitis. Non-cirrhotic portal fibrosis is also increasingly common in HIV positive patients due to the use of certain HAART medications (e.g. didanosine; see Chapter 13).

Arboviruses

Dengue: Transmission is by mosquitoes. Hepatic dysfunction is common. Typically, AST > ALT, opposite to the pattern seen in viral hepatitis. Fulminant liver failure is rare. Treatment is supportive and most patients recover within 2–3 weeks.

Yellow fever (flavivirus infection): Occurs mainly in sub-Sarahan Africa. Transmission is by mosquitos. Most patients have a self-limiting febrile illness but some progress to jaundice and multi-organ failure. Treatment is supportive.

Visceral leishmaniasis (kala azar)

This multisytemic protozoal disease is the result of *Leishmania donovani* or *Leishmania infantum*. Transmission is by sand-flies. Patients present with fever, splenomegaly, hepatomegaly, lymphadenopathy, skin lesions, anaemia, diarrhoea and/or neurological symptoms. Serology (anti-Leishmania antibodies) is diagnostic in >90%. Treatment is with liposomal amphotericin, miltefosine or pentavalent antimony. Mortality is higher in immunosuppressed patients.

Leptospirosis

Leptospirosis occurs following exposure to urine from a variety of domestic and wild animals. Clinical features include conjunctival suffusion, raised creatinine kinase, jaundice with mild transaminitis, renal or cardiac involvement. Serology is diagnostic.

Tuberculosis

Mycobacterium tuberculosis can affect the liver in several ways. Caseating granulomatous hepatitis usually results in a mild transaminitis, although occasionally it can lead to hepatic failure. Obstructive jaundice can occur due to lymphadenopathy at the porta hepatis causing extrinsic compression of the extrahepatic biliary tree. TB therapy can also be complicated by a drug-induced hepatitis (see Chapter 23).

Brucellosis

Sporadic cases occur following ingestion of infected unpasteurised milk. Patients present with fever, hepatosplenomegaly, lymphadenopathy, mild transaminitis and pancytopenia. Treatment is with doxycycline + rifampicin for 6–8 weeks and streptomycin for 2 weeks; 10% will relapse. Q fever caused by *Coxiella burnetii* is rarer than brucellosis, but presents similarly. Treatment is with doxycycline.

Toxins

- Illicitly brewed alcohol, containing methanol;
- Natural contaminants of grain (e.g. aflatoxins; risk factor for HCC);
- Traditional herbal remedies;
- 'Bush teas' (Africa and the West Indies) or contamination of flour with pyrolizidine alkaloids (Afghanistan), predispose patients to hepatic veno-occlusive disease.

Chronic liver disease

All causes of chronic liver disease can also occur in a tropical setting. However, chronic viral hepatitis is often much more prevalent.

Schistosomiasis

Schistosomiasis is a collective name for an infection by one of several species of trematodes. *Schistosoma mansoni* is responsible for abdominal schistosomiasis. The trematode is found in freshwater rivers and lakes in tropical regions in Africa and South America (Map 47.1). Patients may develop fever, myalgia and other non-specific symptoms within a few weeks of exposure, as a result of the worms maturing and producing immunogenic eggs. Chronic infection leads to periportal fibrosis and non-cirrhotic portal hypertension. Patients develop massive splenomegaly and oesophageal and gastric varices. Few studies have evaluated gastrointestinal bleeding in this situation, therefore treatment is recommended as per cirrhotic variceal bleeding (see Chapter 14). Cirrhosis is rare in schistosomiasis, unless patients are co-infected with HBV or HCV. Once a chronic schistosomiasis infection is established, complications such as peri-portal fibrosis and portal hypertension can be prevented with a single dose of praziquantel.

48 Tropical liver disease: hepatobiliary

Disease	Endemic area	Clinical presentation	Investigations + findings
Ascaris		Jaundice, cholangitis or pancreatitis (due to common bile duct or pancreatic duct obstruction)	Worms may be visualised as tram-like structures within the bile ducts on US or MRI. Endoscopically worms are occasionally seen migrating up the bile duct via the ampulla
Biliary flukes (*Clonorchis sinensis* and *Opisthorchis viverrini*)		Obstructive jaundice, cholangitis or hepatomegaly	Hepatomegaly ± intrahepatic duct dilatation. Flukes seen emerging from the ampulla on ERCP undertaken for obstructive jaundice
Fasciola		Obstructive jaundice and/or tender hepatomegaly (Onset 3–4 months after infection during the chronic stage of fascioliasis)	CT images often show transient tracks within the liver, which are formed by the liver flukes. Endoscopically, occasionally flukes can be seen emerging from the ampulla
Hydatid		Chronic pain, abdominal mass, incidental finding, sepsis (superimposed infection) or obstructive jaundice (cyst rupture in to the biliary tree)	Imaging is diagnostic. In cystic hydatid disease multiple daughter cysts are seen within a well-defined circular cyst. Alveolar hydatid often mimics a poorly defined spreading liver tumour
Amoebic liver abscess		Right upper quadrant pain, fever and hepatomegaly	Tender hepatomegaly with liver abscess. Serology is diagnostic

Hepatology at a Glance, First Edition. Deepak Joshi, Geri Keane and Alison Brind.
© 2015 John Wiley & Sons, Ltd. Published 2015 by John Wiley & Sons, Ltd. Companion website: www.ataglanceseries.com/hepatology

As in parenchymal tropical liver disease, clinical history and geographical setting are essential in determining the underlying aetiology.

Solid liver mass

Although the overall differential diagnosis of a solid liver mass remains similar worldwide, variation in risk factors which are associated with certain tumours make some lesions much more prevalent in certain areas.

Hepatocellular carcinoma: HCC is the sixth most common cancer worldwide. There is significant variation in incidence globally; the highest rates are seen China, South-East Asia and Africa. In Africa and South-East Asia, approximately 60% of cases are attributable to chronic HBV infection compared to just 20% in Europe and North America. Targeted HBV population vaccination programmes in these high-risk areas are causing rates of HCC to fall slowly (see Chapter 40).

Cholangiocarcinoma: The highest incidence of CC worldwide has been reported from north-eastern Thailand (96 per 100 000 population compared to 1–2 per 100 000 population in the UK). CC is largely a tumour that occurs sporadically in the Western world but in South-East Asia the exceedingly high incidence is attributed to endemic levels of biliary fluke infestation (*Clonorchis sinensis* and *Opisthorchis viverrini*) and chronic typhoid carriage (see Chapter 41).

Cystic liver mass
Pyogenic liver abscess

Pyogenic liver abscesses have an equal prevalence worldwide. They often occur at more than one site in the liver and are frequently associated with intra-abdominal sepsis (e.g. diverticulosis). Blood cultures and imaging are often diagnostic. In addition, diagnostic aspiration of the abscess are often useful in defining antibiotic therapy. A prolonged course of antibiotics is usually required and resolution is monitored by serial imaging (e.g. repeat US every few weeks).

Amoebic liver abscess

Amoebiasis is the result of an *Entamoeba histolytica* infection. Differential diagnosis includes a pyogenic liver abscess. Treatment is with metronidazole and a luminal amoebicidal agent (e.g. diloxanide furoate). Aspiration is only indicated in the severely ill, large left lobe abscesses (that are at risk of rupturing into the pericardium) or where there is diagnostic uncertainty. When aspirated abscess fluid resembles 'anchovy sauce'.

Hydatid disease

Hydatid disease has two distinct subtypes: cystic and alveolar.

Cystic hydatid disease: Cystic disease is more common and is caused by the tapeworm, *Echinoccoccus granulosus*. Cysts can develop anywhere but 75% of cases have hepatic involvement. Most hepatic cysts are asymptomatic and are found incidentally but they can cause abdominal pain and obstructive jaundice. Imaging is diagnostic; multiple daughter cysts are seen within a well-defined circular cyst. A suspected hydatid cyst should not be aspirated for diagnostic purposes as leakage of contents can cause anaphylaxis or disseminated abdominal hydatid disease. Treatment is with high-dose albendazole for several weeks–months to sterilize the cysts. Larger cysts that remain symptomatic (e.g. biliary obstruction or abdominal pain) following sterilisation are then amenable to percutaneous aspiration–injection–reaspiration or surgical resection. Asymptomatic degenerate parasitologically sterile cysts, with an amorphous centre and calcified wall, do not require treatment.

Alveolar hydatid disease: Alveolar hydatid disease is caused by *E. multilocularis*, found in South America, China and Central Europe. It localises to the liver in almost all cases. Patients present with weight loss, fever, pain and hepatomegaly. Imaging mimics a poorly defined spreading liver tumour. Alveolar hydatid has a much poorer prognosis than cystic disease. Treatment is with long-term albendazole for palliation (although its efficacy has not been demonstrated), radical surgical resection or liver transplantation.

Parasitic biliary obstruction
Ascaris

The roundworm *Ascaris lumbricoides* infects more than 1 billion people worldwide. Occasionally, worms migrate up the biliary tree or pancreatic duct, causing cholangitis, liver abscesses or pancreatitis. The worms can be removed endoscopically.

Treatment is with albendazole.

Trematodes

Biliary flukes: *Clonorchis sinensis* and *Opisthorchis viverrini* are endemic in South-East Asia. Infection leads to obstructive jaundice and cholangitis. Chronic infection is strongly associated with hepatolithiasis (intrahepatic bile duct stones) and cholangiocarcinoma.

Treatment is with praziquantel.

Liver fluke: Fasciola is found in temperate climates and the Middle East. Typically, patients present with obstructive jaundice or tender hepatomegaly. Eggs of the flukes may be found in faeces, bile or duodenal aspirates.

Treatment is with triclabendazole.

49 Nutrition and liver disease

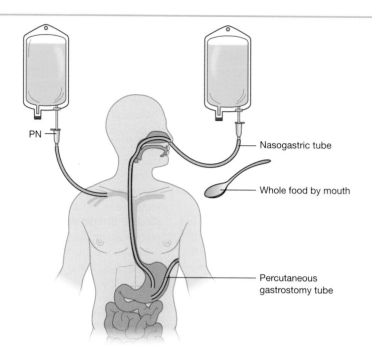

PN

Nasogastric tube

Whole food by mouth

Percutaneous
gastrostomy tube

Figure 49-1 Feeding methods.

Box 49-1   Daily nutrition requirements for patients with cirrhosis

General principles
Energy: 30–35 kcal/kg dry body weight
Protein: 1.2–1.5 g/kg dry body weight (20–30% of daily calories)
Fat: 10–20% of daily calories
Carbohydrate: 50–60% of daily calories
Dietary pattern: where possible avoid unnecessary dietary restrictions, 4–7 small meals/day including a carbohydrate-rich snack before bed
Vitamin and micronutrient deficiencies (e.g. vitamins A, D, E, K, zinc and calcium): screen and correct as necessary
Alcohol: avoid

Specific situations
Ascites: low to moderate sodium restriction – often poorly tolerated
Hepatic encephalopathy (HE): maximise medical treatment of HE (see Chapter 19), do not limit protein intake, and consider branch chain
   amino acid enriched formulae

Malnutrition occurs in 65–90% of patients with chronic liver disease. Despite being a common clinical finding it is frequently under-diagnosed and under-treated. Malnutrition including micronutrient deficiencies can precipitate decompensation and overall nutritional state is recognised as an important predictor of survival in cirrhosis.

Definitions

Malnutrition: a diet that does not provide adequate calories and/or protein to maintain nutritional status. It includes malabsorbtion and over-nutrition (see Chapter 27).
Enteral nutrition (EN) includes:
• Oral nutritional supplements (ONS); and
• Enteral tube feeding (e.g. nasogastric, nasojejunal or via a gastrostomy).
Parenteral nutrition (PN): intravenous administration of nutrition.

Pathophysiology of malnutrition

A variety of mechanisms contribute to malnutrition in chronic liver disease: poor dietary intake, malabsorption, increased protein losses, low protein synthesis, disturbances in substrate utilization, and hypermetabolism (e.g. increased energy expenditure and sympathetic drive as well as insulin resistance). Patients with substantial alcohol consumption often replace meals with alcohol and therefore consume a diet lacking in micronutrients and protein. The effect of poor diet is often compounded by malabsorption due to the toxic effect of alcohol on the small bowel and pancreas. In cirrhosis, hepatic glycogen stores are deplete, gluconeogenesis increased and glucose production low (making patients susceptible to hypoglycaemia). This catabolic nutritional state means protein and amino acids are often used as an alternative energy source leading to loss of muscle mass. When acutely unwell,

Hepatology at a Glance, First Edition. Deepak Joshi, Geri Keane and Alison Brind.
© 2015 John Wiley & Sons, Ltd. Published 2015 by John Wiley & Sons, Ltd. Companion website: www.ataglanceseries.com/hepatology

appetite and intake are reduced and if admitted to hospital, malnutrition is often compounded further as patients are frequently required to fast for clinical procedures (e.g. endoscopy, US).

Micronutrients

In alcoholic liver disease, deficiencies in water-soluble vitamins and trace elements (vitamin B, C, thiamine, zinc, magnesium) are common. Deficiencies in fat-soluble vitamins (A, D, E and K) are prevalent in cholestatic liver disease.

Diagnosis
Nutritional assessment

The Subjective Global Assessment of nutrition is based on the history, examination and/or simple anthrometry (e.g. mid arm circumference), and has been shown to be an effective screening tool to detect malnutrition in liver disease. Recently, the National Institute for Clinical and Healthcare Excellence (NICE) in the UK have recommended that all inpatients are screened for malnutrition using the Malnutrition Universal Screening Tool (MUST):

1 *BMI score:* weight (kg)/height (m²);
2 *Weight loss score:* percentage unplanned weight loss;
3 *Acute disease effect score:* the time over which nutrient intake has been reduced and/or likely to be impaired.

Although this tool can be used in patients with liver disease, care should be taken with interpretation when ascites or oedema are present as the BMI will be artificially elevated. There are specific nutrition screening tools for cirrhotic patients (e.g. Royal Free Hospital Global Assessment tool) but they are complex and time consuming. New simpler screening tools (e.g. Royal Free Hospital Nutritional Prioritising Tool) are currently being developed and validated and may supersede the use of MUST as a screening tool for malnutrition in inpatients with cirrhosis. Blood tests (e.g. serum protein or albumin) are also of limited use in this cohort and studies suggest they are a much better predictor of severity of liver disease than malnutrition.

Nutritional management
Cirrhosis

Patients with cirrhosis are encouraged to eat frequent meals (4–7 per day with a late evening snack). This switches off gluconeogenesis and improves nitrogen economy. Supplemental EN is recommended if patients cannot meet their daily nutritional requirements. In the first instance ONS are recommended, followed by TF if ONS fails or is medically impractical (e.g. HE). Cirrhotic patients are at risk of refeeding, so EN should be started slowly and supplemental parenteral multivitamins and thiamine routinely prescribed. Refeeding bloods including phosphate, potassium, magnesium and calcium, should be checked and replaced parentally as

necessary. Gastrostomy placement is associated with significant risk in this population and should be generally avoided.

Acute liver failure

Nutritional therapy is an important (but not immediately necessary) part of the management of fulminant liver failure. While patients are being medically stabilised hypoglycaemia is a common problem and parenteral glucose administration is often necessary.

Alcoholic hepatitis

EN has been found to be as effective as steroids in treating severe alcoholic hepatitis and has a lower 1-year mortality.

Hepatic encephalopathy

In patients with overt HE, TF should be commenced promptly and is safe, even in the presence of varices. There is no evidence that protein restriction improves HE and it may actually compound muscle wasting. A whole protein or branch chain amino acid enriched formulae is therefore advocated.

Ascites and oedema

Low to moderate salt restriction is recommended in ascites (<6.9 g/day salt). This is achieved by avoiding added salt and pre-prepared meals: patients frequently find this strategy unpalatable.

Osteoporosis

Osteoporosis is prevalent in patients with chronic liver disease. A DEXA scan is advised at diagnosis and should be repeated every few years. Long-term calcium and vitamin D supplements are recommended for prophylaxis.

Transplantation and liver surgery

Optimal preoperative nutritional state has been shown to reduce operative morbidity. Following liver transplantation, normal food and/or EN should ideally be initiated within 12–24 hours.

Intestinal failure-associated liver disease

Liver dysfunction is common in patients with intestinal failure receiving PN. In those receiving short-term PN, liver biochemistry is often transiently abnormal. In patients receiving long-term PN, steatohepatitis and cirrhosis can occur. Liver dysfunction can be managed by avoiding line sepsis, ensuring patients do not receive parenteral over-feeding and encouraging enteral nutrition where possible. Treatment: soybean-based parenteral lipid emulsions are reduced or replaced by lipid emulsions containing medium chain triacylglycerol, mono-unsaturated fatty acids or fish oil. Parenteral choline and taurine supplementation, oral antibiotics and UDCA can also be considered. End-stage IFALD is an indication for small intestine and/or liver transplantation.

Further reading

Aithal GP, Watkins PB, Andrade RJ, Larrey D, Molokhia M, Takikawa H et al. Case definition and phenotype standardization in drug-induced liver injury. *Clin Pharmacol Ther* 2011;89:I806–15.

Bellomo R, Ronco C, Kellum JA, Mehta RL, Palevsky P & Acute Dialysis Quality Initiative Workgroup. Acute renal failure – definition, outcome measures, animal models, fluid therapy and information technology needs: the Second International Consensus Conference of the Acute Dialysis Quality Initiative (ADQI) Group. *Crit Care* 2004;8:R204–12.

Bridgewater J, Galle PR, Khan SA, Llovet JM, Park JW, Patel T et al. Guidelines for the diagnosis and management of intrahepatic cholangiocarcinoma. *J Hepatol* 2014;60:1268–89.

European Association for Study of the Liver (EASL). EASL clinical practice guidelines: Wilson's disease. *J Hepatol* 2012;56, 671–85.

European Association for Study of the Liver (EASL). EASL clinical practice guidelines: management of hepatitis C virus infection. *J Hepatol*, 2014;60:392–420.

European Association for Study of the Liver (EASL). EASL clinical practice guidelines on the management of ascites, spontaneous bacterial peritonitis, and hepatorenal syndrome in cirrhosis. *J Hepatol* 2010;53:397–417.

European Association for Study of the Liver (EASL). EASL clinical practice guidelines: management of chronic hepatitis B virus infection. *J Hepatol* 2012;57:167–85.

European Association for Study of the Liver (EASL). EASL recommendations on treatment of hepatitis C 2014. *J Hepatol* 2014;61:373–95.

European Association for Study of the Liver (EASL), European Organisation for Research and Treatment of Cancer (EORTC). EASL-EORTC clinical practice guidelines: management of hepatocellular carcinoma. *J Hepatol* 2012;56:908–43.

Moore KP & Aithal GP. Guidelines on the management of ascites in cirrhosis. *Gut* 2006;55 Suppl 6:vi1–12.

Papastergiou V, Tsochatzis E & Burroughs AK. Non-invasive assessment of liver fibrosis. *Ann Gastroenterol* 2012;25:218–31.

Runyon BA & Aasld. Introduction to the revised American Association for the Study of Liver Diseases Practice Guideline management of adult patients with ascites due to cirrhosis 2012. *Hepatology* 2013;57:1651–3.

Vilstrup H, Amodio P, Bajaj J, Cordoba J, Ferenci P, Mullen KD et al. Hepatic encephalopathy in chronic liver disease: 2014 practice guideline by the American Association for the Study of Liver Diseases and the European Association for the Study of the Liver. *Hepatology* 2014;60:715–35.

Williams R, Aspinall R, Bellis M, Camps-Walsh G, Cramp M, Dhawan A et al. 2014. Addressing liver disease in the UK: a blueprint for attaining excellence in health care and reducing premature mortality from lifestyle issues of excess consumption of alcohol, obesity, and viral hepatitis. *Lancet* 2014;384(9958):1953–99.

Index

Page numbers in *italics* refer to illustrations

Hepatology at a Glance, First Edition. Deepak Joshi, Geri Keane and Alison Brind.
© 2015 John Wiley & Sons, Ltd. Published 2015 by John Wiley & Sons, Ltd. Companion website: www.ataglanceseries.com/hepatology